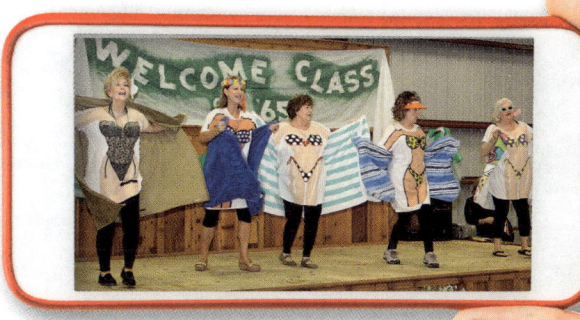

Emily Braddock Jones

2015

Also by Emily Braddock Jones

Love, Laughter & Losing My Keys

Aging Fearlessly

The Good, The Bad & The Awesome

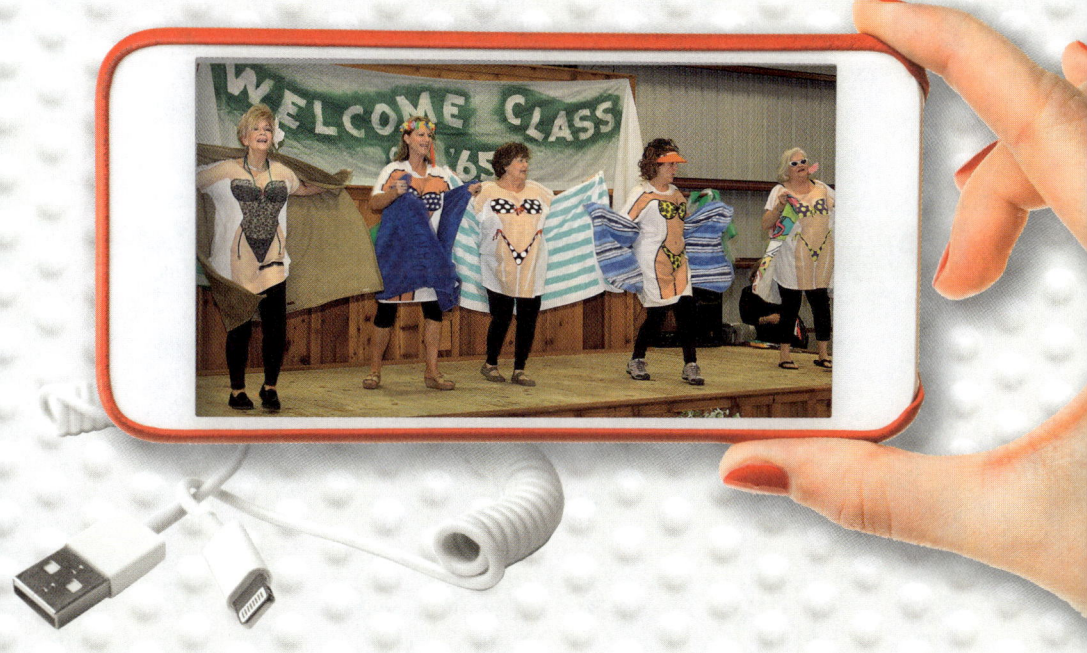

Emily Braddock Jones

CROOKED CREEK PROPERTIES

Library of Congress Control Number
2015911815

Printed in the United States of America

Design and production by Cyndi Clark
Cover photo by Pat Pate
Author photo and chapter opening photos by Leilani Salter (www.leilanisalter.com)
Interior photos submitted by members of the 1965 class at West Point High School

First edition October 2015

Front cover and title pages, from left: Emily Braddock Jones, Marie Portera, Norma Clark Atkins, Barbara Norris Bryan and Ruthie Stafford Weathers perform *Itsy Bitsy Teeny Weeny Yellow Polka Dot Bikini* at the 50th class reunion of the West Point High School class of 65. Classmates were extremely relieved they weren't actually wearing bikinis.

CROOKED CREEK PROPERTIES
www.deludeddiva.com
crookedcreek47@gmail.com

Thanks to the entire class of 1965
at West Point High School (Mississippi).

We have been the cast of characters in the lives
of each other—going from young and foolish
to older and delusional enough to think we are
ageless. It's been a great ride and I wouldn't
have missed it for the world.

Contents

The awesome

Acknowledgments

Many thanks to my editor, Joe Lee, and graphic designer Cyndi Clark for giving this treatise style and continuity. Special thanks to Pat Pate who served as our class photographer and was kind enough to share her shots from our latest reunion. Also thanks to one of my Tribe members, Carole Higgins Morton, who went to the trouble of gathering old photos from our glory days and putting them into a slide show to present during the reunion.

And of course, I would be remiss in not expressing my love and gratitude to the Marganita's, a group of local girls from the Class of 65 who have taken the place of the sisters I never had.

Emily Braddock Jones

Exploring the New Frontier

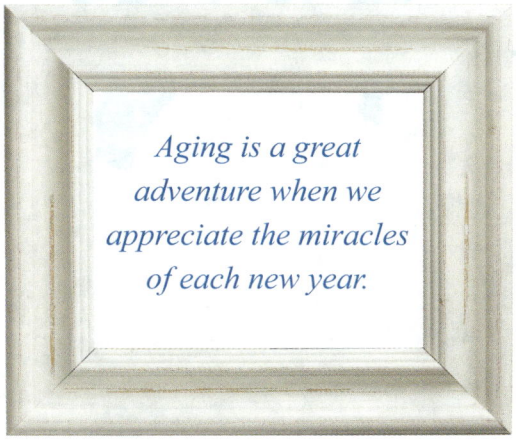

Aging is a great adventure when we appreciate the miracles of each new year.

It is estimated that every eight seconds, someone in America celebrates their sixty-fifth birthday. We have more senior citizens in America today than we've had at any point in history—somewhere around 75 million according to most estimates. If you're there, you're in good company.

Maybe it's wishful thinking on my part, but "old" doesn't look the way it once did. Take a look at Jane Fonda, Helen Mirren, and Christie Brinkley and try to label them with the word *elderly*. You can't do it. My grandmother seemed old at age 55 and I would never imagine her whitewater rafting, hiking the Sipsy, or running a half marathon … which is what my gang was up to at that same age.

Staying "forever young" has become a national obsession since modern medicine and healthier living conditions have conspired to add a decade or two to our life expectancies. That translates into 20 more years of new experiences with hearts pumping, brains churning, and bones carrying us farther and faster than we ever dreamed.

> • • •
>
> "Aging is a mystery cruise to an undisclosed destination in wildly unpredictable weather conditions."
> —From *Goddesses Never Age* by Christiane Northrup, MD

It can be scary, yet mysteriously exhilarating if we have our attitudes and activities focused on the positive column. One observer put it this way: "Aging is a mystery cruise to an undisclosed destination in wildly unpredictable weather conditions."

My childhood friends and I who have formed a sort of "Belligerent Boomers Club" (meaning we're not fading away without a fight) have booked passage on this cruise. We are working hard to get the most from our senior years, and we plan to hold "old" at bay long enough to allow us to evolve into a new breed of senior citizens.

As we attempt to recalibrate our lives to maximize the good things about aging and minimize the bad, we are experimenting with new approaches and attitudes to carry us joyfully into this last big adventure. We have suggestions on what to pack and who to invite as traveling companions. We hope the tips we offer will inspire other Boomers who find themselves on this same adventure; that it will help them persevere on a cold winter day when it would be easier to give up—and give in to the rocking chair.

Aging fearlessly demands more than mere hope that everything will turn out alright. Hope must always be supplemented with "action" to keep the movable parts greased and the brain at full throttle.

We have begun paying more attention to our accruing limitations and figuring out how to work around them. If nothing else, we've learned to laugh at the things that trip us up—the memory loss, the stiff joints, and a plethora of age-related maladies which seep into our fortresses and crack the masonry.

Best of all, we share our courage to move deeper into the new frontier. Maybe you will be inspired to join us after hearing our story, which began way back in 1947 and continues to this day. Our secret? We celebrate anything and everything and are continually adding items to our collective bucket list. We simply don't have time to get old right now—and I don't see it happening in the foreseeable future.

Here's to your age, whatever it is! Just remember, age doesn't matter unless you are a cheese ... or a bottle of fine wine.

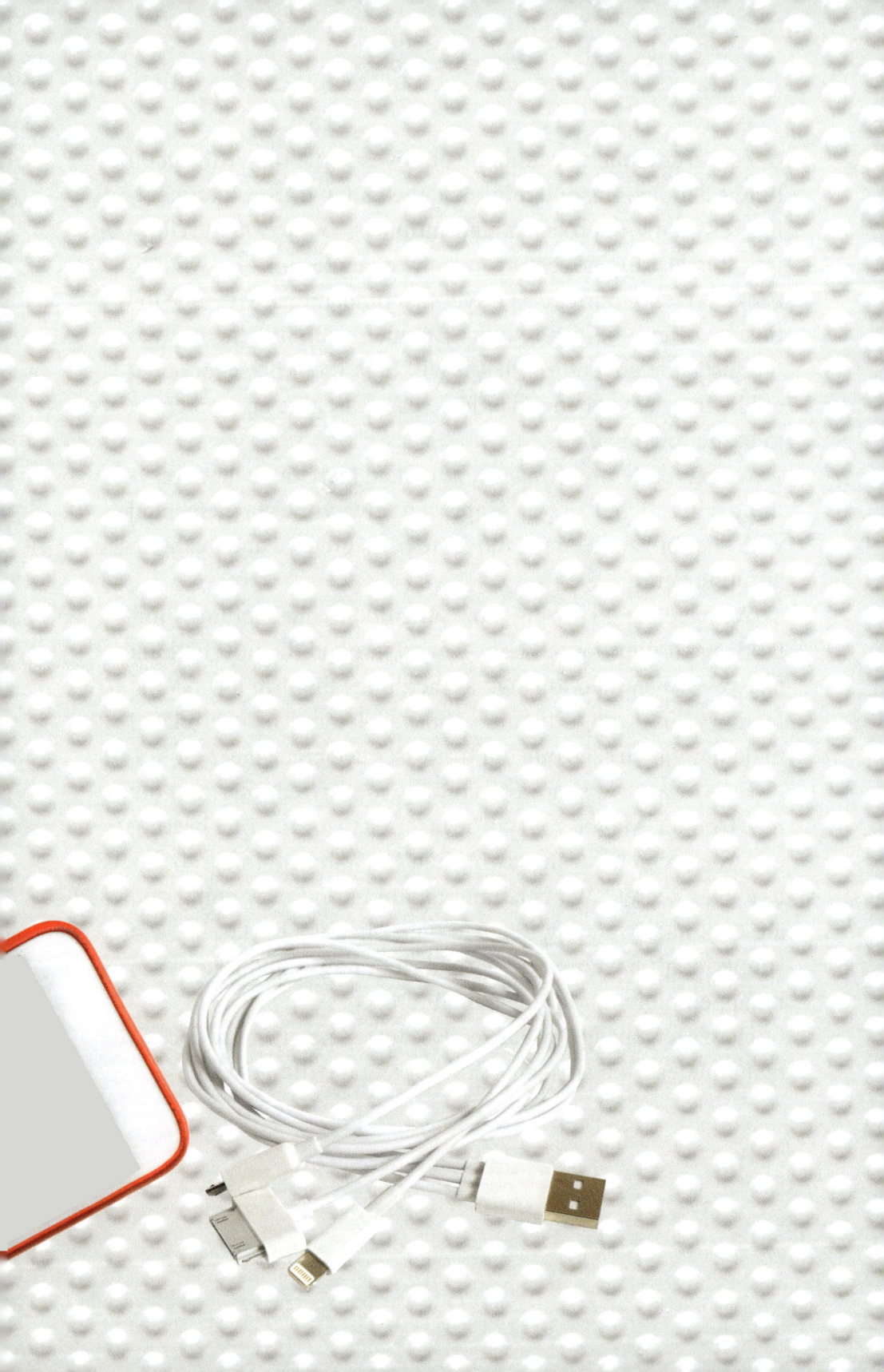

The Good

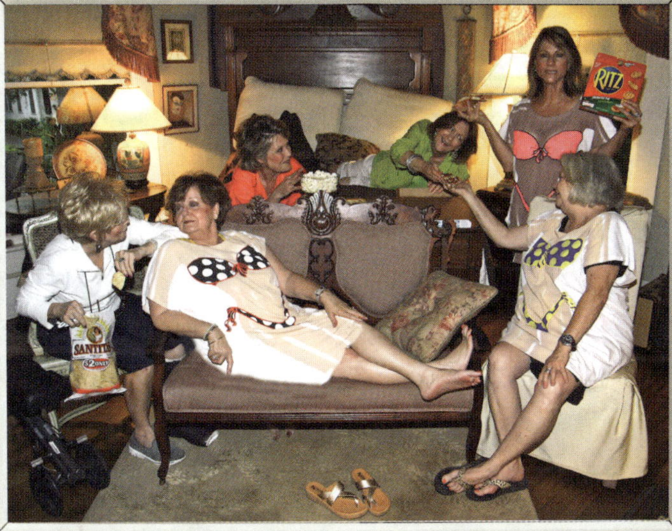

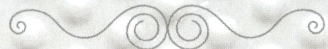

Acting like kids again is the perfect solution for aging.
For a little while we are 16 again and we still do sleepovers.

Back row, from left: Brenda Montgomery Chambliss, Barbara Norris
Bryan and Marie Portera (standing). Front: Emily Braddock Jones,
Norma Clark Atkins and Ruthie Stafford Weathers.

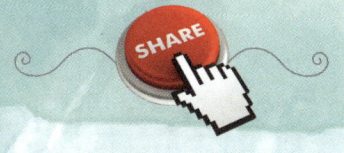

Curtain Call for the third act

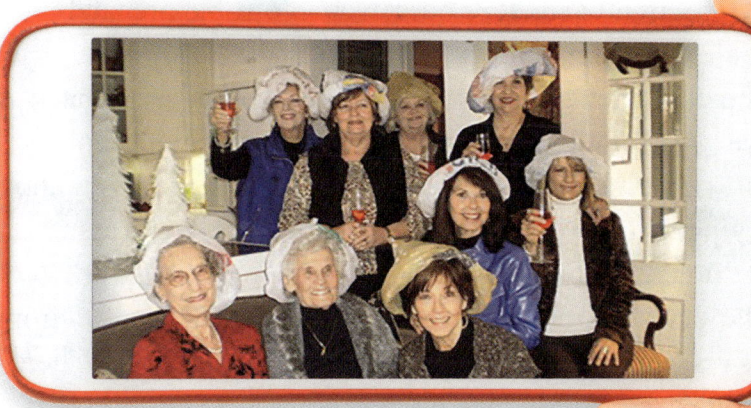

On our 60th birthday we wore bags on our heads
and found them quite stunning.

All of us over the age of 50 have something to look forward to that eluded our ancestors. We get another life to live. No kidding. You heard it here.

A recent study reveals that people in the twenty-first century get an extra 34 years added to their life expectancy. That's practically another lifetime, which affords us the ultimate do-over!

Yippee! I love do-overs, since I rarely get it right the first time.

If you're a part of the Baby Boomer generation, you have just been born again. Hallelujah! Can I get an AMEN?!? Let's get it right this time, shall we?

The old way of thinking suggested that we were born, peak somewhere around the middle ages, then begin the spiraling descent into decrepitude. The NEW paradigm suggests the last three decades of life aren't all that different from childhood, when we were feisty, inquisitive, and full of ourselves.

Then along came puberty and we got all hung up on our insecurities and struggles to be part of the cool crowd. All the while we tried to squeeze ourselves into some prenatal mold our parents dreamed for us.

The third act gives us an opportunity to circle back to where we started and reinvent ourselves without concerns about what others think. At last, we can be ourselves without worrying that we will look naïve or stupid. Like Picasso once said, "It takes a long time to become young."

The entire world operates on a universal law of entropy that says everything is in a state of decline and decay. There's only one exception to this universal law—the human spirit. It allows us to keep growing and developing into who we were intended to be. It just takes some of us longer than others.

Act III calls for nourishing the spirit with wonder and delight in doing what we love. It requires daily doses of laughter and a lot of prayer. Without prayer we don't have a prayer of succeeding in our third act!

And speaking of laughter, I had a personal experience I will carry with me for those times when my enthusiasm for the aging process is missing. I awoke one morning feeling depressed and frustrated over some little thing. I called one of my sons in tears and he listened, then reported that he had just seen a guy over on Highway 82 wearing a pair of panties on his head.

All the pent-up frustration finally had an escape hatch. I laughed so hard I had to lie down on the bed. What a day-changer that little story was! I wish I could find the guy and thank him for helping me put my troubles in perspective. If you see me walking down the street with a pair of panties on my head, you'll know I'm just trying to spread a little cheer. That, or I've finally gone and lost it and don't know which end to put the panties on.

> • • •
>
> "The very act of thinking and behaving as if you are in your prime actually reverses the physical decline."
>
> —From *Goddesses Never Age* by Christiane Northrup, MD

The curtain call for Act Three is somewhere around the sixtieth birthday, which we should celebrate (rather than wringing our hands and considering ourselves over the hill). To be over the hill suggests that we are past our prime and growing so rusty we cannot do anything exciting or meaning-ful any longer. I prefer to think of it as "near the peak," and that we can do pretty much whatever we please.

We can eat dinner at 4 p.m. and our most embarrassing secrets are safe with our friends because they can't remember them for more than 20 minutes. No one expects us to run into a burning building or be last in the buffet line—age before beauty is a beautiful concept. Your supply of brain cells is finally down to a manageable size, and I've learned from experience that it's not a good idea to give yourself a haircut after three margaritas.

That quote by Dr. Northrup has given me a new lease on life as I climb ever higher on the ladder to heaven … at least I hope that's my happy destiny. It suggests that I don't have to age if I don't act like an old person. In other words, fake it until you make it. I can do that.

The new rules of engagement

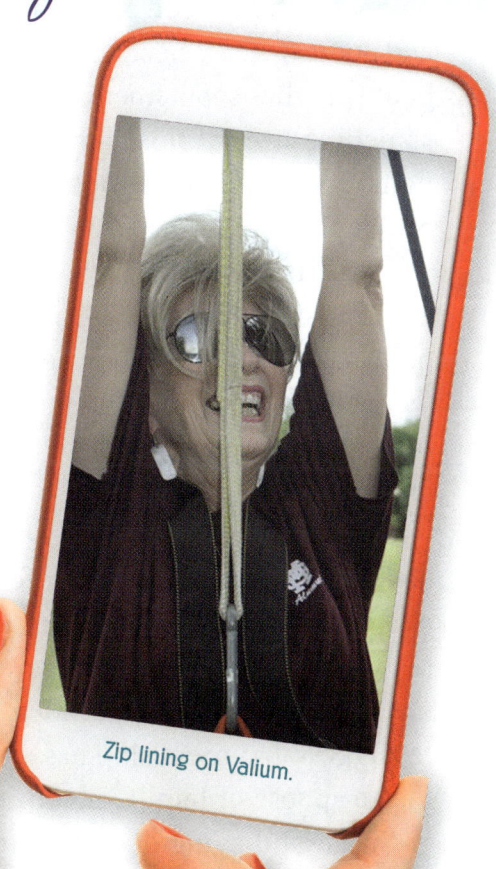

Zip lining on Valium.

I was catching up with my friend Marcia at the supermarket this week and she asked what my new book will be about. I said it will offer ideas on how to approach the aging process from an angle other than just letting my generation's itinerary fade away without a fight.

"Aging," Marcia almost spat in disgust. "I'm against it," she said unequivocally, as if discussing the H1n1 swine flu. She was in peak condition and had just come from her Pilates class. This girl wasn't going lightly and I liked her spunk.

Hey, it just occurred to me that most of my "research" for the new book is conducted at the supermarket. I wonder if my groceries are tax deductible as a business expense.

All this talk about aging piqued my growing fascination with what factors conspire to put one senior citizen on jet skis and another in a wheelchair. We can turn to doctors, self-help books, herbal supplements, costly creams, and surgeries, but sometimes we overlook a powerful weapon that could help us fight illness and depression, speed recovery, slow aging, and prolong our lives: our friends.

Our friends are the ones who rush to help in times of crisis and who can laugh with us into the wee hours as we share our personal adventures. They are the ones shuffling beside us as we make our way through the Baby Boomer's last frontier— old age. Just remember, age doesn't matter unless you are a cheese or a bottle of wine. Or did I say that already?

Several years ago the *American Journal of Public Health* had a Harvard research team follow 16,000 men and women over age 50 for six years. The results showed a clear connection between being socially active and involved, and preserving memory and cognitive abilities. There is increasing evidence to suggest that friendship has an even greater effect on health than a spouse or family member.

Successful aging does not mean that we never experience adversity in our lives. Knees do wear out and need replacing; arteries clog and need mending; eyesight and memory fades;

hearing just up and leaves—a plight curiously common to the male population.

It dawned on me that aging can be a funky sort of fun as long as you have a sense of humor and someone to share it with. It's kind of like dancing—you can do it alone but it's so much more fun with a partner.

• • •

"Many people die at twenty five and aren't buried until they are seventy five. Admittedly, aging is a profoundly personal and self-directed activity. To age successfully suddenly seems a hero's journey of mythological proportions. It calls for improvisation, creativity, and a wicked sense of humor when all else fails."

—Emily Jones & Benjamin Franklin
(Obviously not during the same century)

If aging were a team sport, my team would have the ball about now. So far, we're having a good game. So what do I consider successful aging? It's obviously NOT the maintenance of perfect health or even the absence of disease. It's not avoiding pain and suffering, frailty or vulnerability. Maybe it's simply living our lives to the fullest of our capacity to do so for as long as we continue to breathe.

Benjamin Franklin is credited with saying, "Many people die at twenty five and aren't buried until seventy five." Admittedly, aging is a profoundly personal and self-directed activity. To age successfully suddenly seems a hero's journey of mythological proportions. It calls for improvisation, creativity, and a wicked sense of humor when all else fails.

My personal game plan is called *The Five Rules of Engagement*. It is now on sale for $19.99 on the Home Shopping Network, but—today only—I give you a rough outline free of charge. It goes like this: In my house there are five rooms. They are labeled 1) spiritual (my personal faith practices) 2) physical (the icky exercise and diet), 3) environmental (home and garden) 4) fiscal (staying ahead of the tax collector) and 5) social (sharing experiences, hopes, dreams, and laughter with like-minded people).

A good day for me requires that I visit all five rooms, if only to air them out. Otherwise, life can get dangerously out of balance and aging can slip in while you're looking the other way.

Lately my "physical room" has been sadly ignored. But hark, A New Day Cometh and many ills can still be undone. So come on, you kids of the 40s, 50s and 60s—let's get our game faces on and thumb our noses at this aging thing. And aging gracefully is certainly not my goal. There's nothing graceful about it unless you're a fictional character. So go ahead and age as disgracefully as you can. It will be lots more fun.

Miracles, metaphors, and magical moments

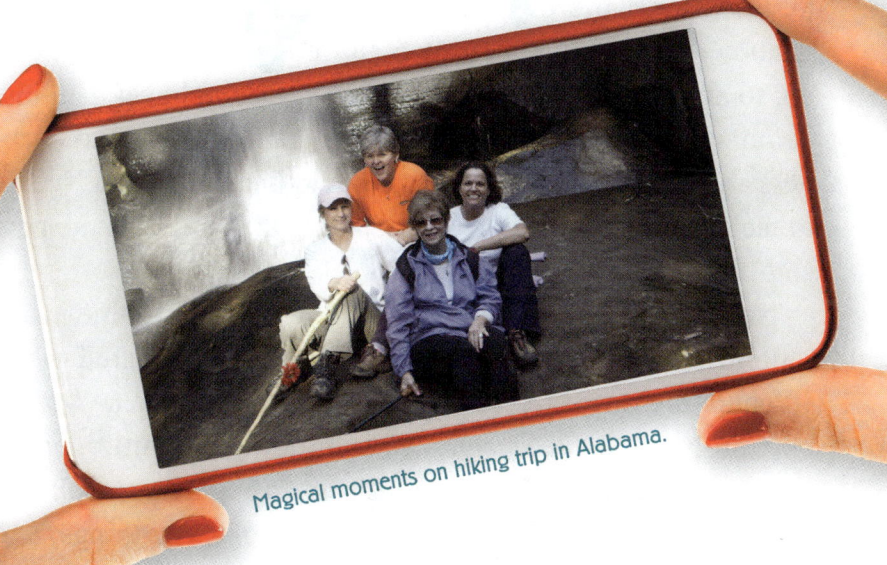

Magical moments on hiking trip in Alabama.

With the arrival of each season, I renew my commitment to exercise and diet. That typically occurs after an extended vacation when diet and exercise have been blown—due to weather, illness, or maybe just a "staycation" when you take a break to refill your tank.

My recent staycation turned out to be downright painful in the end because I was stabbed by guilt every time I saw someone power walking or jogging by my house. Why wasn't that me, I wondered? Because, you lump, you've been glued to three seasons of *House of Cards* which came with your Netflix service. Of course, the series demanded a steady supply of microwave popcorn so I wouldn't have to miss a single moment cooking, cleaning, or breathing fresh air.

Then I discovered that a bag of M&Ms tossed into the popcorn created a nice juxtaposition of flavors and I was destined for a life of what we once called the "shut-in"—a chubby one at that. I went two entire days without connecting to another human being, not that I'm proud of it. I'm just demonstrating how quickly someone can descend into darkness and become a post. Sitting is addictive and adding Netflix to the mix can be deadly. (You did hear that sitting is the new smoking, right?)

Needless to say, I was in need of a tune-up and some inspiration to get back on track. It miraculously appeared when I found my fifteen-year-old copy of *The Spirited Walker* by Carolyn Scott Kortage. The subtitle of this little gem is *Fitness Walking for Clarity, Balance*, and *Spiritual Connection*. Hmm. Obviously I didn't have any of those things, and I wanted them!

Armed with the promise that miracles will emerge with each spirited walk if combined with mindfulness and meditation, I laced up my shoes and headed out the door before the sun rose. I was excited about my very first spiritual experience/workout and full of expectations. As instructed, I mumbled "I am here, I am here" with each step until I passed Everett Kennard's house. Sitting on the porch and hidden by the shrubbery, Everett yelled, "Good morning, Emily. Who's that you're talkin' to?" I turned fifty shades of purple, and from then on I practiced my mantra silently—lest I be thought a crazy woman.

> • • •
>
> "There are only two ways to live your life. One is as though nothing is a miracle. The other is as though everything is a miracle."
>
> –Albert Einstein

As I picked up the pace, I looked all around me for the miracles. Would I see a message from God in the clouds, a diamond in the gravel road over behind the Baptist Church, or what? It took me exactly 48 minutes to discover that the miracle was that I had showed up, dressed out, and actually enjoyed myself. Instead of mulling over my problems (complicated by the sad state of the world), I began to notice the little things—the beautiful ferns on a porch on Washington Street; a newly-restored vintage smokehouse on the same street; the arrogant body language of a big ole tabby cat (who was clearly unimpressed with my effort). I made a mental note to get some ferns and stop obsessing over what a cat might think of me.

I didn't see any jaw-dropping miracles, but I did see a bird sitting high on a rooftop singing his heart out for no particular reason. I saw a monarch butterfly flitting from flower to flower sampling the nectar for free.

Albert Einstein once said, "There are only two ways to live your life. One is as though nothing is a miracle. The other is as though everything is a miracle." I choose the latter. If it was good enough for Albert, it is good enough for me.

I guess the real miracle will be if I can motivate myself to repeat the process tomorrow.

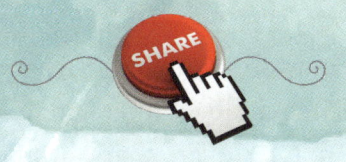

The underused art of the compliment

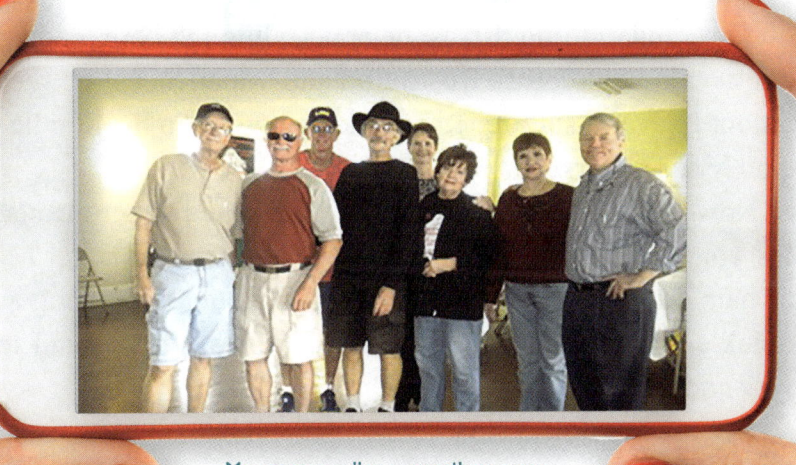

My gang can live a month on one good compliment.

It has been said that a human can live for two months on a good compliment. Me? I can go a week, tops, and then I start fishing for them.

How long since you paid someone a genuine compliment? And more important, how long since you received one? In this world of war, pestilence, and ridiculous gas prices, maybe it's time we spent our compliments more freely instead of hoarding them silently. The results could change the course of a day for someone, and maybe even spark a chain reaction which could change the world. It sure couldn't hurt.

As I stood in line at the Piggly Wiggly, I was fuming below my normally cool exterior with a fake smile pasted on my face. There I stood with two cans of Alpo Filet Mignon dog food (the only thing Her Highness Lucky Dawg will eat). Ahead of me was a harried-looking lady with 22 items in her cart—and we were in the express lane which clearly stated 20 ITEMS OR LESS! Couldn't she read, better yet count?

That kind of thing drives me crazy, although I am reading a book on how to defuse frustration and impatience with meditation. I haven't succeeded at making it work in the middle of a busy supermarket.

Now to the compliment part. I just wanted to set the stage for you: the rule-breaking lady had the most beautiful head of hair I'd ever seen on a woman. It was thick and long and twinkled with auburn highlights as she tossed her head this way and that while unloading the cart.

I've always wanted to toss my hair, but hairspray is a mixed blessing. On one hand it holds your hair in place; on the other hand it holds your hair in place. It makes your "do" impervious to high winds, tornadoes, or cyclones. There's no hair tossing in my world.

Without any thought of worming my way ahead of her, I felt compelled to pay this woman a compliment. I caught her eye and blurted out what I'd been thinking, and a 150-watt smile miraculously transformed her face in an instant. She glanced down at my pitifully few items and stepped aside so I could go ahead of her.

Wow, this compliment thing really works. But seriously, I wasn't being manipulative—it was a genuine compliment. Usually I secretly admire something about a stranger but keep my mouth shut. Why do we do that? Complimenting people doesn't cost a penny. Why not "brighten the corner" when we can.

> • • •
>
> As Southerners, we learned at an early age we can get away with chatty, catty criticism as long as it's accompanied by those three little words: BLESS HER HEART. I've blessed so many hearts I should receive my very own clerical collar.

Let's suppose you're at a large gathering and you spot someone you admire for some little thing. You tell your companion, "Charmaine looks great today, doesn't she?" We'll say that to whomever we're standing beside … unless we're standing beside Charmaine, who will never know how great she looks.

But let Charmaine commit some wardrobe infraction and we gleefully whisper that Charmaine's Crocs don't do much for her lace skirt. This is okay as long as it's tagged with the words BLESS HER HEART. As Southerners, we learned at an

31

early age we can get away with chatty, catty criticism as long as it's accompanied by those three little words. I've blessed so many hearts I should receive my very own clerical collar.

Today I challenge you to pass out a genuine compliment. Just be aware that good intentions *can* go awry, such as with comments like, "You look good for your age." I call these *complisults*.

We've all gotten them from some thoughtless acquaintance who makes an offhanded comment about you that makes you smile, and then go, "Wait … what? Hey!" My all-time favorite (which I've heard on more than one occasion) is, "Wow! You're a lot smarter than you look!" I'm working on my look, but then I was born with it and the chances of my looking any smarter are slim to none.

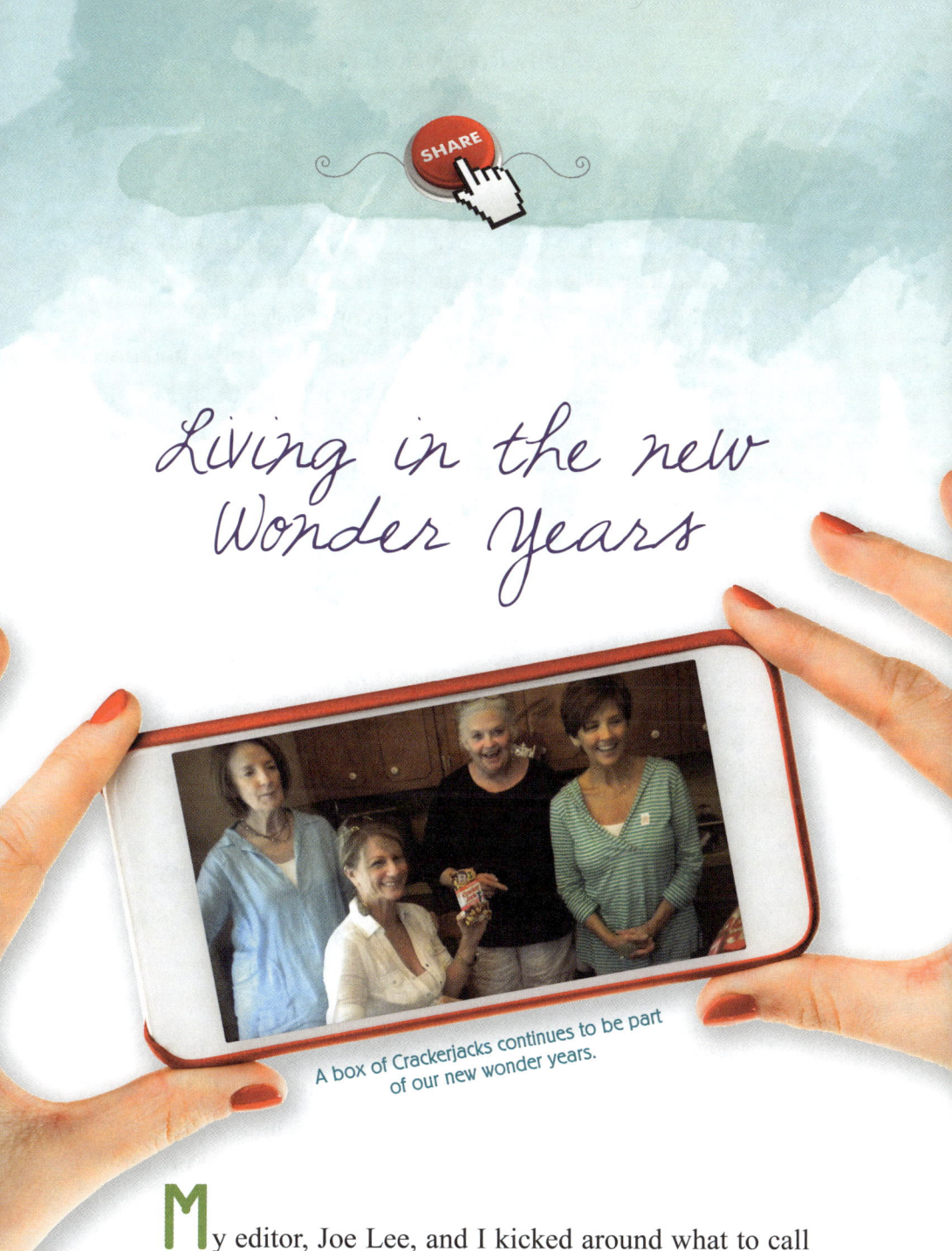

Living in the new Wonder Years

A box of Crackerjacks continues to be part of our new wonder years.

My editor, Joe Lee, and I kicked around what to call this book. I wanted to call it *The Wonder Years*, but he felt it might be confused with the television show by the same name which had a good run about 25 years ago.

Truth be known, my crowd has been waking up in the wonder years for the past decade. You wonder where you parked your car, what you had for lunch, and you have to check to make sure you remembered your underwear.

Last weekend seven of my high school girlfriends (and one brave boy) celebrated our matriculation into an unspeakable age which no one ever said out loud. It was too painful to admit we had become upper-class senior citizens—trying to plan our 50th class reunion, no less!

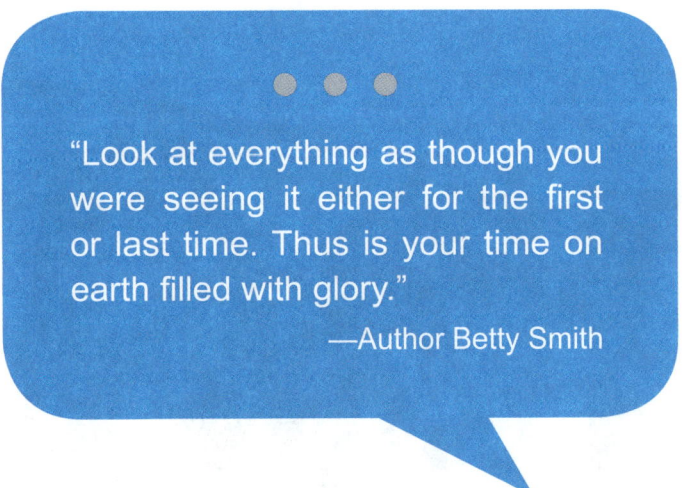

"Look at everything as though you were seeing it either for the first or last time. Thus is your time on earth filled with glory."

—Author Betty Smith

No way. Couldn't be. Denial was hovering above our heads like hungry mosquitoes. We tried in vain to swat them away but they persisted. So we did what we did a half century ago when our parents were bugging us: we planned even more outrageous activities.

Today we are faced with a brand new set of challenges. And cataracts, arthritis, bad knees, high blood pressure, clogged arteries, and even cancer aren't going to rain on our parade.

As pals forever, we've finally opened our hearts to each other the way we never would have dared 50 years ago. We share our hopes and dreams without fear of judgment. We embrace what is, even if it's become one size too large and know without a doubt these people have our backs—forever. There are no words for feelings like these. Friendship and love are much too shallow.

We whooped it up and acted like we were 12 for a while. Without parents to shut us down we blossomed into tiger lilies. We recalled growing up in the greatest small town ever chartered without air conditioning, computers, cell phones, and only one TV in the house (which transmitted only six hours a day).

Back in the day, we were forced to find other outlets for our energy. We had fun long before Facebook or "pudding pops" (I think it's an internet game), and it's so much more satisfying to have honest to goodness, face to face fun.

We weren't pretending at all this weekend. We really were 12 again as we spread a little gossip and complained about the boys in our class who have suddenly become good (and very handsome) men. We agonized about women's clothing in the twenty-first century. I had just purchased what I thought was a dress and it turned out to be a tunic. That would certainly turn heads if I wore it in public—but not in a good way.

Funniest thing, we had also developed a deeper side which made us tear up at the spectacular sunset over the lake and become giddy looking at a cornfield across the road. Wow ... they've been there all along, and it was as if we'd never seen them before.

We had come full circle. We met in a playpen while our doting mothers and grandmothers looked on. Today we ARE our grandmothers who have all gone to the Great Hereafter. Thank goodness we still have each other to wander around with in the NEW wonder years.

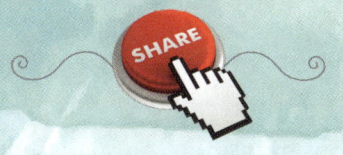

Happy days are here again

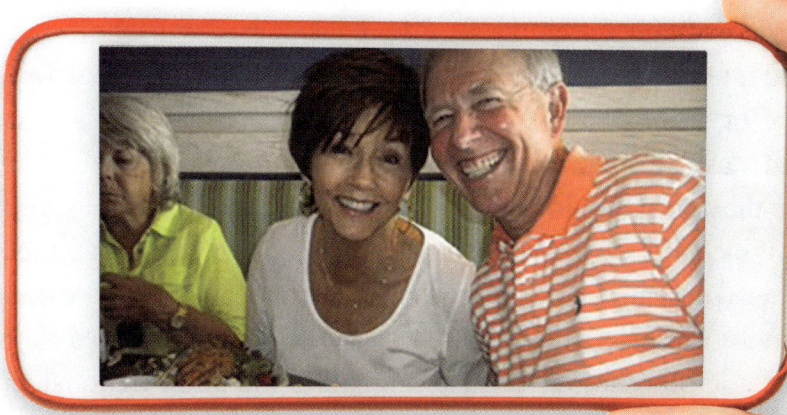

Food and friends forever.

Happy days are here again—caffeine and chocolate are in! It seems to me that my palate has grown more discriminating the older I get. The freckled-faced girl who thought eating an asparagus spear was as close to torture as it gets … now can't get enough of them. Ditto for avocados and kiwis (which I thought for the longest was in the insect family).

But wait. Enter the food police, who are constantly changing dietary recommendations on us so often that we get whiplash.

I spent the entire decade of the 1980s limiting myself to one cup of coffee per day, which made me irritable, not to mention so drowsy I shouldn't have been allowed to operate my hair dryer. Instead of salt I used something that tasted like a cross between a science project and rat poison (well I haven't actually tasted rat poison, but that's what I imagine it would taste like). Now a panel is studying the notion that a little salt on the table might actually be healthy!

Surprise, surprise, the guvment now admits they got it all wrong telling us cholesterol and fat cause high cholesterol and fat thighs. The panel is now encouraging us to knock back five or more cups of Joe, which will make our minds sharp and stave off dementia and maybe even diabetes. Well, what are they going to do about us conscientious folks who listened to their caffeine warnings and 30 years later can't remember where our car is parked or even what make and model we are driving? What do you have to say for yourself, Uncle Sam, and you bloody food Nazis? It's your fault, and I'm considering legal action.

Then there's the incredible egg, which was considered a product of the devil himself. Thankfully I ignored the rule to limit my egg consumption and made up for my caffeine deficiency with omelets, quiches, and deviled eggs (which is probably how that dish got its name). Either I lived through it or I'm among the walking dead.

Yes, Henny Penny, the sky is no longer falling and you can begin spitting out eggs like a gumball machine. And to the little Morton Salt girl (now a 104-year-old woman), you can take off your raincoat and get in your rocking chair. The sun is out and salt is okay again—well, if your doctor says so.

The new demon of the day is sugar. Yeah, well, I wonder how many years it will take for the food police to reverse that ruling and issue a statement calling for daily servings of Ding Dongs and GooGoo Clusters. I wouldn't be surprised if they decide decades down the road that tobacco cures blindness and eating magnolia leaves will reduce racism.

> ● ● ●
>
> "Delight is a crucial ingredient in agelessness. Ignore the food police. Indulge your appetite for the pleasures of food shared with good company … in peaceful contemplation of the fruits of the earth."
>
> —From *Goddesses Never Age* by Christiane Northrup, MD

All this focus on diet and being told what we should and shouldn't eat is beginning to get on my nerves, and it's sucking the joy out of eating. One of life's great pleasures used to be when families and friends would gather around the dinner table and savor recipes passed down from grandmothers and great grandmothers. No one cared what was in the delectable dishes, and we lapped up to-die-for casseroles made with that other science project called margarine. We now learn margarine is tragically hydrogenated, another no-no for your table.

Yay, bring on the butter, girls, real *buttah!* Happy days are here again. And don't forget to keep your kitchen clean and eat out often.

"We were not designed to eat alone watching bad news on television," declares Christiane Northrup, author of *Goddesses Never Age*. "We are creatures who seek connection, and when we sit down to enjoy a meal together, our differences melt away. The emotional bonding allows us to rebuild our tissues and organs with a sense of love and belonging."

That, my friend, is why my little band of soldiers in the war against aging does a lot of eating out together. And trying new restaurants is a healthy pastime after all.

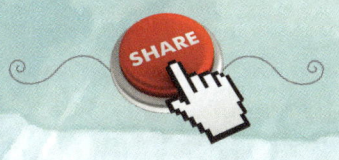

Stop aging gracefully.
Try aging gratefully instead!

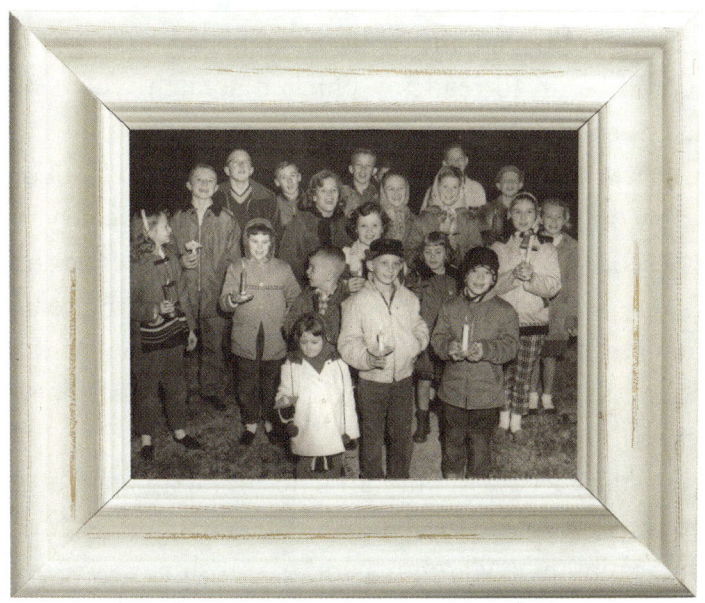

Once we were carolers, now grateful to be caroled to.

Years ago, I began keeping a daily journal. Frankly that's just a pop culture word for *diary*. Hardly a day goes by that I don't use that journal to rant about what needs ranting about and listing all the small miracles (a.k.a. blessings) that are embedded in each day.

At first, I bought expensive, leather-bound blank books in which to record my observations, and the things I wrote were designed to make me sound like a cross between Martha Stewart and Ann Landers.

These days I just pick up a cheap black and white composition book and fill it up each month with the bold, unvarnished truth.

Side note: I have a friend (Putt, are you listening?) who has sworn, upon hearing of my demise, to get to my house pronto and get those journals to the landfill. I cringe to think someone would read the tedious maniacal diatribes—as if they could begin to read my chicken scratch where no T is crossed nor I is dotted.

I love it when the new month rolls around and I can begin a fresh new book. I especially love the first day of every month, which escorts in hopeful and lofty resolutions equal to New Year's. I typically select a theme for that month. For example, January always accompanies a new healthy diet with plans to lose that pesky ten pounds by Easter. (To date, it has never happened.)

In February I vow to bury all hateful, judgmental attitudes, and be the demure loving person I was meant to be (that lasts about 45 minutes). March ushers in a fresh new season and I begin my spring cleaning with the promise of purging my life of three unwanted items each day. By the end of the month, I just open a box of toothpicks and toss three away.

Well, you get the idea. No point in putting undue pressure on yourself.

November is ALWAYS the month of gratitude. We should

be forever grateful to the dear soul who came up with Thanksgiving—the greatest concept ever devised. It promotes family, food, and an abiding faith in something other than ourselves. Turkey and cornbread dressing, mashed potatoes with gravy, sweet corn, pumpkin pie, and sweet potatoes mashed with brown sugar. The family gathered around the dining room table and football on the television are how we make some of our best memories. (And we gain back the ten pounds we've worked to get off since January.)

> "Every day, offer thanks for the rough spots in life. When you come out the other side, they never look so bad. If you can't be content with what you have received, be thankful for what you have escaped!"
>
> —Emily B. Jones

Incidentally, Abraham Lincoln is the soul most often credited with establishing the Thanksgiving holiday. He lost eight elections, failed twice in business, and suffered a nervous breakdown before being elected president. Certainly we ordinary citizens should be able to muster up a little gratitude.

But back to the journal. I highly recommend the practice of unloading all your feelings—especially the grateful ones—into a little book, rather than boring your friends with the stuff. Even minor disasters have a way of working themselves out when you bring them into sharper focus in your journal, which is your secret confessor and memory keeper. As they say, confession is good for the soul. And my soul is white as the driven snow until it gets peed on from time to time.

Imagine what would happen if you made gratitude your focus for the whole entire year. Not only will it change your life, but the lives of everyone around you.

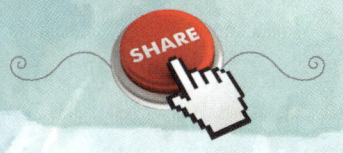

Kick up your heels!

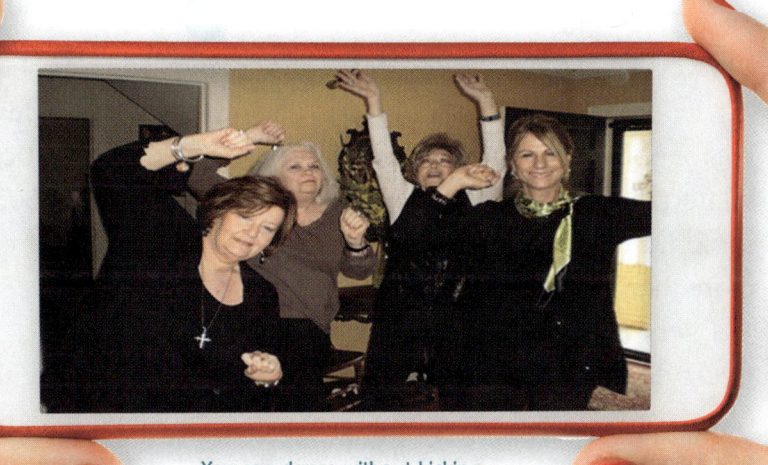

You can dance without kicking,
you know.

Picture it. Several hundred of your best friends from a half century ago are gathered at your high school hangout to relive the best times of your life and pay tribute to one special classmate who left us much too soon.

We lost Gary without any warning when his heart just

stopped beating one day. And it was a big heart. I'm reminded of a note I saw carved on a headstone in my family cemetery in North Mississippi: "Death leaves a heartache no one can heal; love leaves a memory no one can steal."

Classmates from around the country flew in to pay tribute to Gary. It was an impromptu class reunion none of us had prepared for. The majority of us had put on a few pounds, and there was more silver hair than I remembered—if there was hair at all. The faces were a little more lined by years of laughing, smiling, and breathing. It didn't matter one iota because with each new arrival, the years fell away and we were 16 again.

Everywhere you looked, folks were group-hugging. I got so carried away I planted a big kiss on some guy I later learned was sent in by the power company to check a dead outlet. No matter; it's amazing how your inhibitions fade away about the same time as your eyesight (and your ability to hear out of more than one ear).

Everyone was on the dance floor performing some sort of freestyle dance maneuver as we tried to keep pace with the tunes we loved 50 years ago. You could dance with a guy for a moment, then turn and dance with a girl whose name you couldn't quite recall. Suddenly six or eight of us would join arms and pretend we were the Rockettes until we were breathless. Some were doing *The Twist* while others were sliding and twirling in a failed attempt to mimic *Dancing with the Stars*. I glanced around to see if anyone had thought of having an EMT on hand.

After 50 years, The Torquays (our high school dance band) had reunited to carry us back to the 1960s—only better. Gary had been the lead singer in recent years and his brother, Jeff, came to take his place for one last tribute concert. In the old days, I would have been sitting in the corner wrapped up in all my teenaged insecurities, both praying for and dreading the moment when a guy would come over to ask me to dance. It would be embarrassing to be a wallflower … and even more horrifying to put yourself out there to try to demonstrate some kind of rhythm.

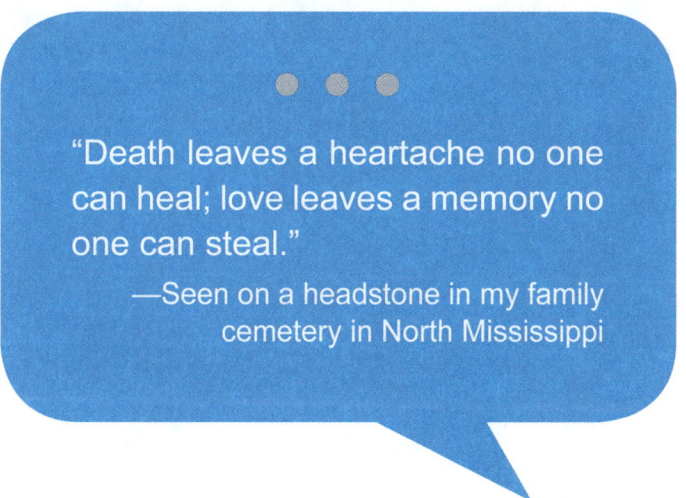

"Death leaves a heartache no one can heal; love leaves a memory no one can steal."

—Seen on a headstone in my family cemetery in North Mississippi

The band broke for a moment to let us catch our breath and pass around the blood pressure cuff. An old boyfriend came over and commented, "I see you still have no rhythm. You were zigging while everyone else zagged." Well, I never! Until that moment, I thought I had perfect rhythm. I thought I was one of the cool kids. At least I tried, posing for hours in front of the mirror trying to look aloof yet rhythmic at the same time.

Then I recalled how exhausting it was to appear cool and aloof while all the uncool kids were whooping it up on the dance floor, oblivious to how ridiculous they looked. I think that's called *fun*, and what a shame it took me 50 years to figure it out. These days my old gang gets together to lose that unhealthy sense of self and become absorbed by something larger and more inclusive.

> • • •
>
> Having fun is a lot of work, but so is anything that produces priceless memories you can pull up anytime … especially on those cold winter days when issues of aging seem overwhelming.
>
> —Marie Portera, Class of 65

Did I detect a bit of childlike glee moving through the room? It was extremely contagious. Suddenly the band broke into *(You Make Me Want To) Shout* and everyone was on their feet joining the pack of gyrating senior citizens who were kicking their heels up, throwing their hands up and tossing heads back while singing "yeah yeah, yeah yeah" until we worked ourselves into a frenzy. (Our children would have nightmares for weeks if they could have seen the spectacle).

"Having fun is a lot of work," commented my friend Marie, "but so is anything that produces priceless memories you can pull up anytime … especially on those cold winter days when issues of aging seem overwhelming."

Suddenly it all made sense. Being cool doesn't take us very far in this life, and it alienates us from our fellow creatures with whom destiny has ordained that we shall live out our existence on this earth. Lucky us. No, I mean it … LUCKY US … until the morning after, when we tried to rally to watch some Mississippi State football. My left hip didn't seem to work anymore and everyone was hoarse from singing, no make that *shouting*.

I've said it before and I'll say it once more: Aging is a team sport, and not so bad if you have someone to do it with. You are finally free to enter a sort of second childhood where no one cares if your socks don't match, and *getting lucky* means you found your car in the parking lot. And best of all … you can be yourself and your friends will love you anyway.

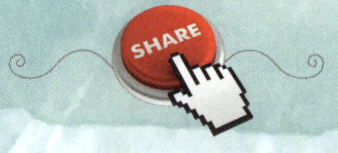

Age with open hearts and minds

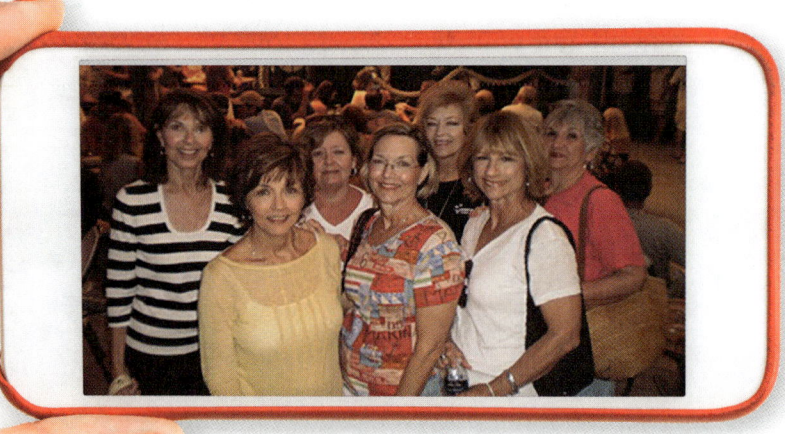

… and always dress up when you go barhopping!

Up until recently I approached this aging thing with dreams of rainbows and unicorns, and I tried chasing shadows and demons away with pixie dust and optimism. Life just doesn't always cooperate and sometimes the messy conditions can overwhelm us.

My son, William, called my bluff on some of my hypocritical attitudes the other day when I was complaining about Microsoft introducing new software. "It will require users to learn a whole new set of rules and procedures when using the internet," I complained. Stomping my foot, I added, "I don't have the capacity nor the desire to learn."

> • • •
>
> "As a wise old man once said, 'Do what you can about what you can and don't worry about what you can't.'"
>
> —Daddy Scott, my friend and Murrah's granddaddy

I was livid and gave the company a verbal thrashing with a string of naughty words. William took one look at me and casually noted that people only get old *when they refuse to consider new ideas and reject new ways of doing things.* Uh-oh. I think I aged 20 years under his cool, accusing stare.

Okay, so I will try to open my mind—but only a crack, mind you. I don't want the few brains left to fall out.

I believe most of the resistance older folks have to new ideas is fear-based; we wring our hands and watch helplessly as our world slowly slips away. Only when we choose to live and let live do we set ourselves up to remain forever young.

The minute we identify with the rest of mankind (rather than insisting on the tired "us-against-them" approach), we can relax and enjoy the ride.

Since the beginning of time the world has been continually changing, and we would be wise to do what we can to keep up.

Aging is not lost youth, but a new stage of opportunity to stay in the game even though sometimes we don't feel like it. It's often tempting to run and hide when time is pounding at us and we lose friends and family members who have shared our disappearing world when it was at its peak.

We lose a little piece of that world with each loss, but a big chunk can be reclaimed on a single evening when my child-hood friends get together, kick off our shoes, and reflect on the good ole days.

Find serenity in the midst of chaos

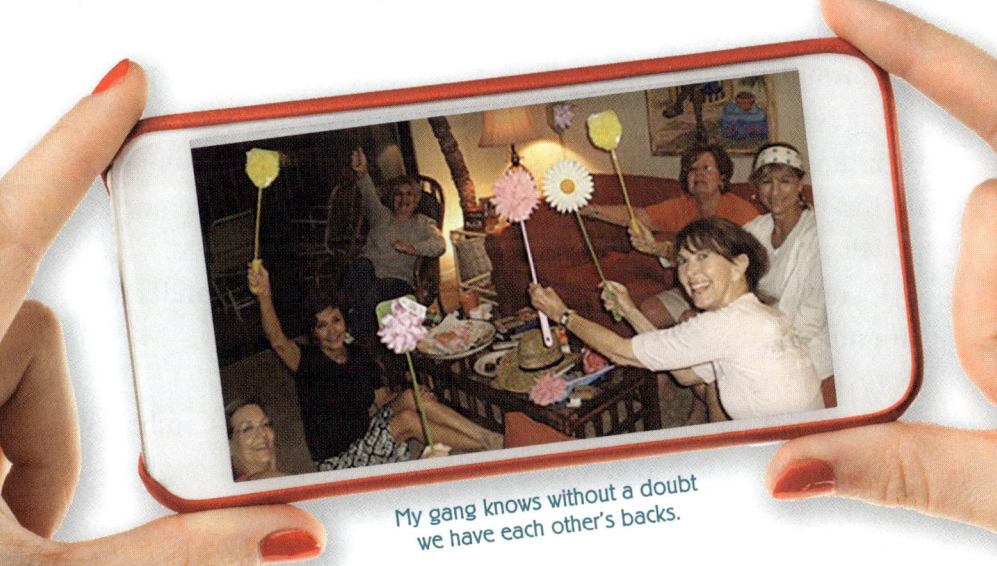

My gang knows without a doubt
we have each other's backs.

The news ... what a bummer it has been lately.

Most days the news alarms us, angers us, and makes me want to go back to thumb sucking. Yet I've stumbled onto the key to restoring a little peace and joy in my days, despite the streaming reports of unspeakable acts going on around the world.

I toss out my system for your consideration, waiving the $19.99 fee I'll be asking on the Home Shopping Network. (Doesn't everything cost $19.99 these days?)

Step One: Cut off what my daddy calls "the idiot box" (television set) and tune in some music—doesn't matter what kind. Some days it's Mississippi Delta Blues. On others it may be Giuseppe Verdi or Gregorian chants. And, naturally, every day will include an ample supply of 50s and 60s tunes to which I sing along word for word. (It helps if you don't have an audience.)

Through divine intervention, I decided to make some changes along my once-frazzled path through life. It seemed to pull me along kicking and screaming. I felt like the caboose on the train to hell, bumping along the tracks without much power to do anything about the rocky ride.

Upon arriving at some questionable destination, I wandered around like a modern day Henny Penny shouting "THE SKY IS FALLING" to anyone who would listen.

The solution to all this *awfulizing* is so simple it's embarrassing. I wish it had not been so long in getting through to me. It goes like this: every action we take is either a victory or a defeat on the road to becoming who we were intended to be. Every single thing we do or think moves us toward our dreams ... or further away. Funny, that simple truth escaped me for six decades.

The process works like this: I eat a chocolate donut for breakfast and I'm backing up. I have a boiled egg and flax seed toast and I'm moving forward. I pull on my Skechers and take a three-mile walk and the sun peeks from behind the clouds. I blow it off because it's too hot, and the sun slips back behind the clouds and I eat two bags of salty potato chips.

> • • •
>
> "Restore and maintain order around you and you'll feel order in your soul. Create beauty around you and you'll feel beauty in your soul, and the magic will magically return."
>
> (This little note to myself was found in a rarely used teapot. I think it is telling me to clean up the house when chaos reigns.)

Maybe I'm critical of someone for some perceived slight or imagined impropriety and I go straight to jail without passing "go." If I look for something positive about that same someone, though, I feel a lot better about myself and that person seems friendlier the next time I see him or her. Weird, isn't it? It's like they sense my secret feelings about them.

Most surprising of all, I found that good-heartedness—or wanting the best for our peers—has the greatest rewards. I knew all this since the day my Sunday School teacher told me about The Golden Rule, but I got distracted and confused power with joy and peace. There really is no relation between the three, you know.

I've also come to believe there's a creative possibility attached to every situation, no matter how dire. Growing older makes us appreciate our youth like we never did when we were in the middle of it. Being ill pushes us to live healthier lives and treasure every day as an opportunity to do everything possible to make it better than yesterday.

And consider this: everything good was likely conceived in the middle of chaos. If we hadn't been forced to beat our clothes on a rock to get them clean, the washing machine might never have been invented. If our forefathers hadn't been forced to wear fig leaves, we probably wouldn't have haute couture to coax us into pulling out our credit cards much too often.

It's a messy world, but maybe if we keep our little corner neat and peaceful, our neighbors around the world will follow suit. If chaos is a necessary step in the organization of our universe, then I am well on my way to a little piece of heaven on earth.

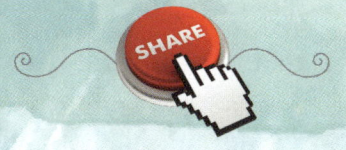

Connected at the hip

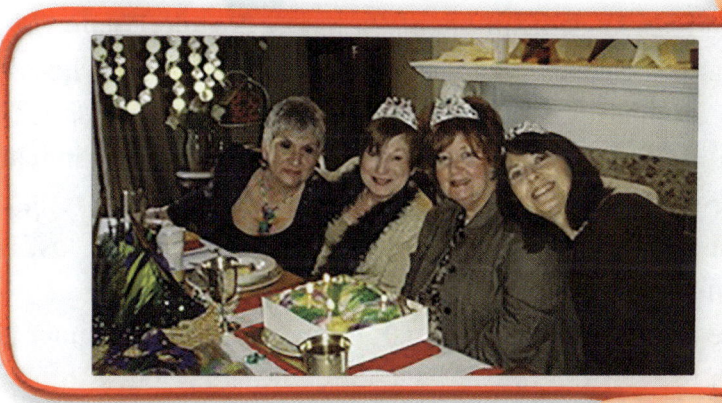

No cellphones in sight while we are eating or celebrating.

ell phones have finally replaced old Ma Bell's home-style clunkers, and even this dinosaur has finally ditched her landline in favor of a smart phone (which is way smarter than its operator).

I haven't begun to learn all its uses, but by the time I'm 70 perhaps I'll be able to turn on my porch light before I get home from a party and deactivate my burglar alarm so I don't wake up all the neighbors at 2 a.m. That's only happened once in the last two years (the staying out until 2 a.m.) and NOT the setting off of the burglar alarm. That happens all the time because I can't remember all the security codes and secret passwords necessary to function in twenty-first century America.

I'm also horrible about keeping up with my cell phone, which is rarely in my hip pocket. I've lost it in the bed covers, underneath the sofa cushions, and I once left it in a shopping cart at Walmart. I've left it at the beach, in Norma's car, and once while riding a rollercoaster—where I also lost my lunch.

A lady in Wisconsin opened a bag of Ripple Potato Chips and started eating. She wasn't looking at the bag when she reached in and felt something hard. It was a cell phone. The blue and silver Nokia contained a T-Mobile SIM card in it and grease stains on the outside. The lady was offered a replacement bag of chips but passed, explaining that she'd lost her appetite for chips for the time being.

The bad thing about losing your phone is that the finder has access to your entire life—which could come back to haunt you in a day or two when they find all the selfies you took while trying to check a side view of your hair.

Personally, I feel cell phones can be an invasion of our privacy. In the old days you could just get in your car and drive around town to escape having to tell anyone what you're up to. Now they can hear the machine running as you slip off to purchase a milkshake after swearing you would never indulge again in this lifetime.

Computer technology has progressed to the point where we can practically poach a perfect egg and have Eggs Benedict waiting on your table for Sunday brunch. And cell phones get more streamlined with each passing model. They used to be the size of a debutante's handbag and came in a suitcase (we called them Car Phones). Now they are small and thin enough for you to slip in your hip pocket, sit on them, and pocket dial Aunt Emma, who listens in on your entire conversation with whomever is riding with you.

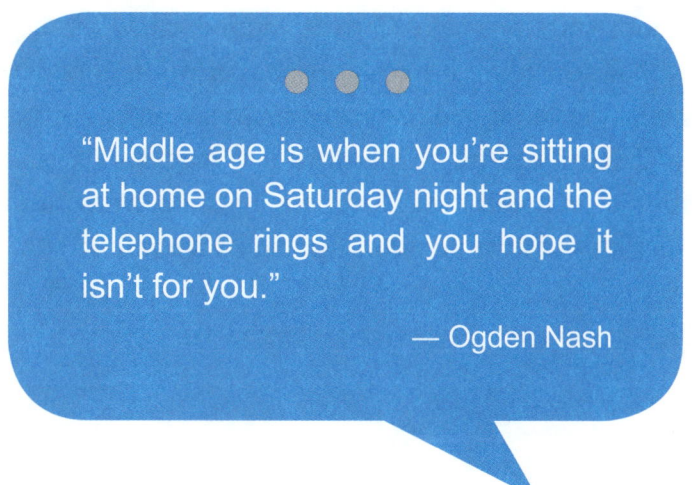

"Middle age is when you're sitting at home on Saturday night and the telephone rings and you hope it isn't for you."

— Ogden Nash

Any day now someone will produce a phone we can have embedded in our wrists so all we have to do is tap to talk. That would certainly reduce the number of misplaced and lost phones. I wonder how many folks have left their "smarty pants" cell phones in their pockets and washed and dried them along with the blue jeans. Cell phones don't like that.

I'm reminded of the late Don Foster, my old friend, co-worker, and sportswriter—who placed his phone in cold storage and we couldn't reach him for days. While unloading his groceries he accidentally placed the phone with the broccoli and oranges in the fridge's vegetable bin. We were trying to contact him about a glitch on the sports page, but the vegetables flatly refused to take the call.

And who hasn't been horrified when they forget to silence the thing and it rings in church? Everyone looks at you like the dunce you are. I can embarrass myself on my own, thank you very much.

And for heaven's sake, don't take calls while you are dining with friends … unless you are awaiting arrival of your organ transplant. And never have private conversations in a public place. I had to endure a two-hour conversation conducted by a lady who was assigned the seat next to me on an Amtrak trip to New Orleans recently. I was trying to read a book, and with her droning on about everything and nothing, I read the same page 43 times and still couldn't grasp its meaning!

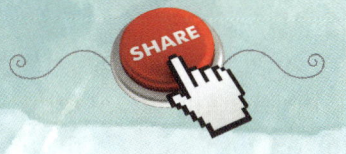

Hope in a bottle

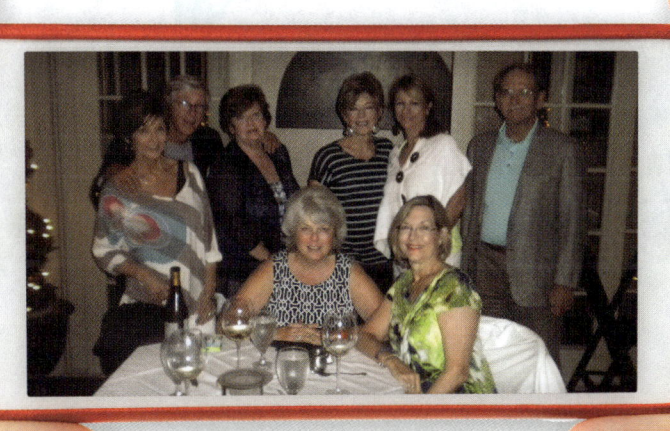

We certainly don't feel like age 70 is nipping at our heels—one of many trips to visit classmates.

A reader dropped me a note suggesting that I do a column slamming cosmetic companies for using thirty-somethings to advertise products these kids won't be interested in for another two decades. Amen, sister. I'm on it.

To be honest, this has been bothering me for some time.

Like for the last twenty years, when I've been completely available to help advertise the fountain of youth. I could be the "before" model on one side of the TV screen, and the peaches-and-cream, twenty-something beauty could be the "after" on the other side.

Just now, there on the big screen in all her dewy glory, is a girl—practically a toddler—smiling glibly while the voiceover describes some miracle cure for wrinkles, feathery lips, thinning hair, under-eye circles, and age spot concealers.

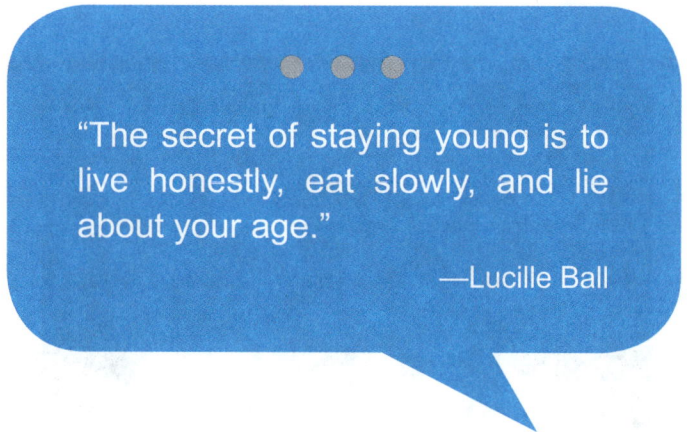

"The secret of staying young is to live honestly, eat slowly, and lie about your age."

—Lucille Ball

Who are these teeny boppers prancing around in their skivvies, advertising foundation garments to lift those parts that won't be sagging for another twenty years?

Judging from the products advertised on the 5:30 nightly news, I figure senior citizens are the only people still tuning in at that time. I'm kind of tired of ads for incontinence, impotence, insomnia, and indigestion. Then there's my favorite: the couple holding hands from separate bathtubs on a beach. Will someone please explain this to me?

Why do we need to look younger anyway? Why can't we

just look our age? There's so much angst about aging that no one seems to feel comfortable about being any age over twenty-one. I'll never forget my fortieth birthday … I received a dozen dead roses and a walking cane with spray mace in the handle. Eighty maybe, but forty?

How do we respond to a comment like "Sixty?!? You don't look that old!" Is that a compliment or an insult? I'm not sure.

Look, age isn't a bad thing. It's a good thing. Age gives summer foliage its rich golden-red hues in the fall. Age gives pewter its rich patina. Age gives cheese its exorbitant price tag. And I once spent three days beating an oak chest with a chain to give it that "aged" look. As people, we get to age without any effort at all.

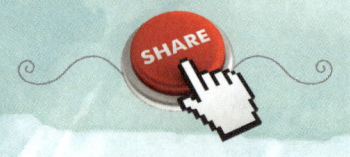

Think big, act small, ward off "The Feebles"

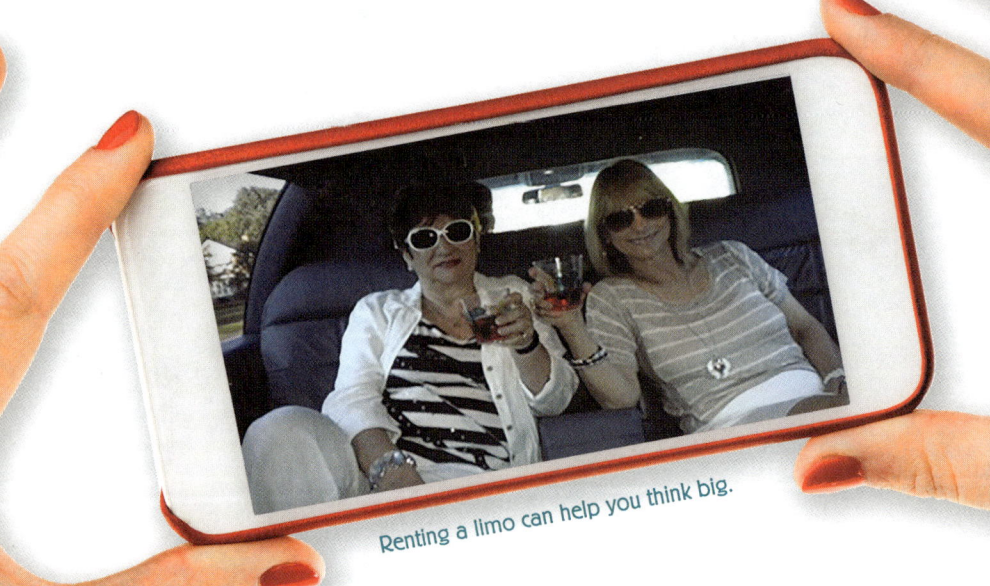

Renting a limo can help you think big.

I've always been a bit of a dreamer. Even as a child, daydreams occupied most of my thoughts while I was supposed to be engaged in other things—like math class, long-winded Sunday sermons, and scoldings for lack of attention during the aforementioned activities.

To this day I don't know how to figure percentages, and I was employed in the banking field for fifteen years. As far as I know, no one was ever the wiser, but then no one ever asked me to perform mathematical projections. I had Dumb Blonde down to an art.

This week I've been pondering the tasty little gems I gleaned from my new favorite author, Julia Cameron, in her book *Finding Water*. This little dissertation is packed with a wealth of suggestions on how to experience smooth sailing in a turbulent world while bringing your dreams into tighter focus. (At my age, tighter anything interests me.)

Faced with mounting global problems which seem hopeless, Cameron suggests we cling to the small and positive steps we can take each day—like walking the dogs, folding the laundry, washing the car, and playing with the cat. (Yes, this self-proclaimed dog lover has adopted a stray cat. She's been living with us for six weeks and still doesn't have a name except Cat. Actually Lucky Dawg, a very competitive female poodle, calls her Crazy Cat.)

But back to mindless activities: Their beauty is that they give you time to let your mind wander to glorious (albeit mostly unattainable) heights. Sometimes I dream of becoming the Editor-in-Chief of *Southern Living*. Other times, when I'm feeling especially delusional, I imagine winning a seat in the U.S. Senate and drafting creative bills to solve America's problems to the extent I'm awarded the Nobel Peace Prize.

See what I mean? You can think as big as you like, so long as you take small steps in that general direction. I renewed my lapsed *Southern Living* subscription and was delighted to learn that the Senate gets more than three months of vacation each year. I'm appointing my exploratory committee to examine my potential political future.

Julia offers some exercises to perform each day. Numero Uno: make a list of the things you love. My list goes on for almost four notebook pages and includes such things as growing a juicy red summer tomato, spotting a rare snowflake falling from heaven, the first crisp cool day of fall, a good book by the fire, and a bubbling pot of chili on the stove. I love the crunch of gravel under my feet while walking in the countryside, hearing the clunk when I shut my car door, and the satisfaction of a clean, orderly home which I hope someday to achieve. (I'm sixty-something and it hasn't happened so far.)

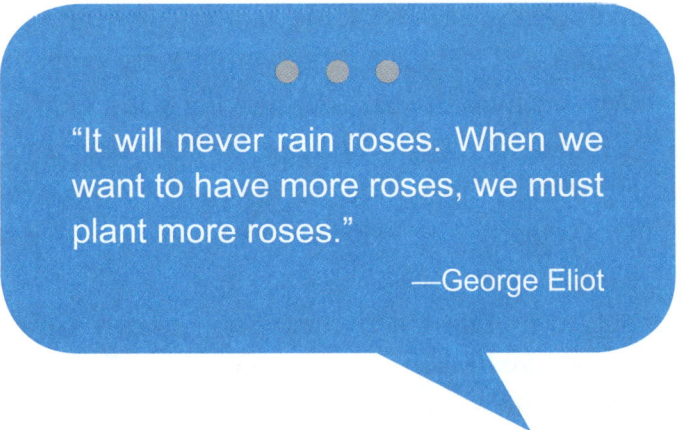

"It will never rain roses. When we want to have more roses, we must plant more roses."

—George Eliot

Oh, and I love to say the word *cockamamie* because it makes me laugh.

This exercise is especially helpful when you are being pushed to the edge of an imaginary cliff and trying to regain your mental footing. Doing the small, doable things can restore a sense of stability during any setback, and a small dose of joy can help you relocate your wandering focus on your ultimate dreams.

In Cameron's book, there is a reminder that if we will simply remain in forward motion even in troubled times— taking insignificant but positive steps toward our dreams—we will eventually achieve the dream that once seemed so elusive. In the words of George Eliot: "It will never rain roses. When we want to have more roses, we must plant more roses."

Or, on Mrs. Cameron's instructions, at the very least we can dig a hole and amend the soil a bit. Maybe the *most* least thing we can do is find the shovel!

It's fascinating how one positive action generates another and another, so taking action becomes the key step in accomplishing something meaningful in this world. Before long, I'm watering a perfectly beautiful rose bush.

All this talk about action carries the hope of warding off that dreaded condition I've begun referring to as "The Feebles." It develops around age 65 for some and 85 for others. I'm going for the upper end.

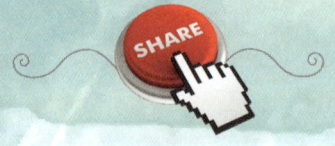

Lucky enough to live past our prime

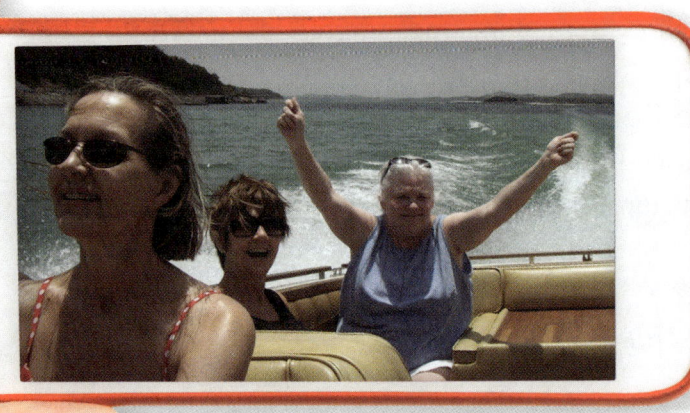

Our prime can change, depending on who we're with on Lake Travis in Austin.

Recently I bought a birthday card for folks born in 1947, the very year I showed up; one of the first to launch the Baby Boom. In the card was the innocuous reminder that life expectancy for babies born at that time was a mere 62 years of age.

Wow. How dare we defy those odds? It dawns on me how much living our forebears missed out on because their lives were cut short. In contrast, my Boomer friends and I are way past that young mark of 62, and we're still dancing badly and kicking up our heels if we can get a brief recovery period.

We are still young enough to travel to faraway places, hike miles on a Saturday, and share our hopes and dreams into the wee hours. We are very much alive, but aware dark forces are lurking and waiting to slow our progress.

> • • •
>
> "As we move from day to day, we realize we can ride the spiral but we cannot harness it. We can put ourselves in charge of some of that process; nature is in charge of the rest."
>
> —From *Inventing the Rest of Our Lives* by Suzanne Braun Levine

Of course, if I had my druthers I would have been born in 1975 and barely turning 40 right now when I could still read the telephone book. Now, there's no real need for a telephone book, and I couldn't read that teeny-tiny type if my life depended on it. One thing is for sure: if I had known I would live this long I would have taken better care of myself.

Our generation has been maligned as the most self-centered, self-seeking, self-interested, self-absorbed, self-indulgent, and self-aggrandizing generation in U.S. history.

Hey, wait! Hold on a minute. Not all of us were draft-dodging, toke-smoking, free-loving, bra-burning hippies who are out to steal our children's financial future and destroy our planet. How can anyone blame that on an entire generation that barely spans 16 years?

Some of us got married, raised families, worshipped in the churches of our choice, held down jobs, and volunteered tirelessly for community projects. We fell into bed at the end of the day then got up the next morning and did it all over again. We did the best we could with the information we had.

If I must, I can apologize for enjoying my time on the planet, but I don't think my generation is any worse or better off than any other. I am a retired bouncing, baby boomer. So, go around me, you yuppies (or millennials, or whatever you are), but please don't glare at me in your rearview mirror.

The magic of the kitchen timer

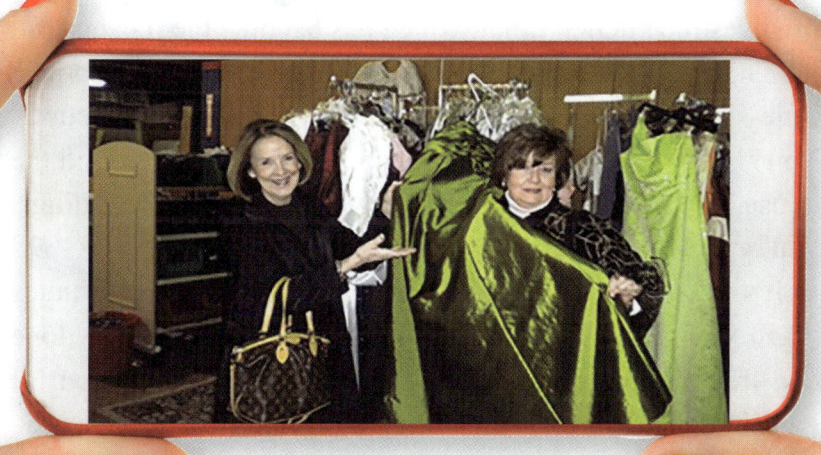

Boogie scooting can also be
performed while shopping

If it's true that cleanliness is next to godliness, then I've been consorting with the devil. But I'm becoming a changed woman who has figured out the key to a happy, well-organized home.

When I was still engaged in a career outside the home, I kept a passably tidy place. For one thing, I wasn't around to mess it up and there was a certain amount of urgency about straightening up each morning. Saturdays were spent on marathon sessions of mopping, dusting, and vacuuming. Bummer.

Since retiring, I have become a world-class procrastinator. I now have all day to get the place cleaned and shined, so I put it off as long as possible. Inevitably, something more exciting comes along and housekeeping is shoved to the back burner. My platform has unabashedly morphed into WHY DO TODAY WHAT CAN WAIT UNTIL TOMORROW?

Then I heard about Boogie Scoots and was intrigued. It involves the kitchen timer, which has become the most useful item in my collection of useless kitchen utensils. I read about a little-known sport called the "Fifteen-Minute Boogie Scoot." You simply set the timer for fifteen minutes, scoot around the house, and clear it of clutter and dust. When the timer dings, you quit. Mission accomplished.

It's amazing what you can accomplish in fifteen minutes when you're totally focused. When time is up, you're done and free to get to the fun stuff. However, nine times out of ten I find that I'm on such a roll that I wind it back up and do another boogie scoot.

It also helps to have a little soundtrack going in the background. Some days it's a Gregorian chant, but more often it's Keb Mo singing the blues.

This also works for small tasks like cleaning off your desk. When the stack of stuff gets so high you can't find your computer, simply apply the boogie scoot. Don't worry about finishing—you can do another scoot the next day or the next. Before you know it, you've got a clean desk with important papers neatly filed away.

This week I took the timer out into the garden, where those fifteen minutes really flew by. If I do only two boogie scoots a day, that amounts to three and a half hours a week! Had I tried to do all that cleaning at once, I would have been overwhelmed (and probably dead from a heat stroke).

> • • •
>
> I read about a little-known sport called the Fifteen-Minute Boogie Scoot. You simply set the timer for fifteen minutes, scoot around the house, and clear it of clutter and dust. When the timer dings, you quit. Mission accomplished.

I'm saving up for the Talking Chef Kitchen Timer. When the time's up, a little voice shares witticisms like WHATSA MATTA WIT YOU? WHY YOU FEEL SO SAD? IS YOUR COOKING THAT BAD? Another message: YOUR OVEN HAS TWO SETTINGS—TOO SOON and TOO LATE. Note: I usually use the TOO LATE setting, and everything comes out toasty. But my house is tidy and life just works best in those conditions.

The Bad

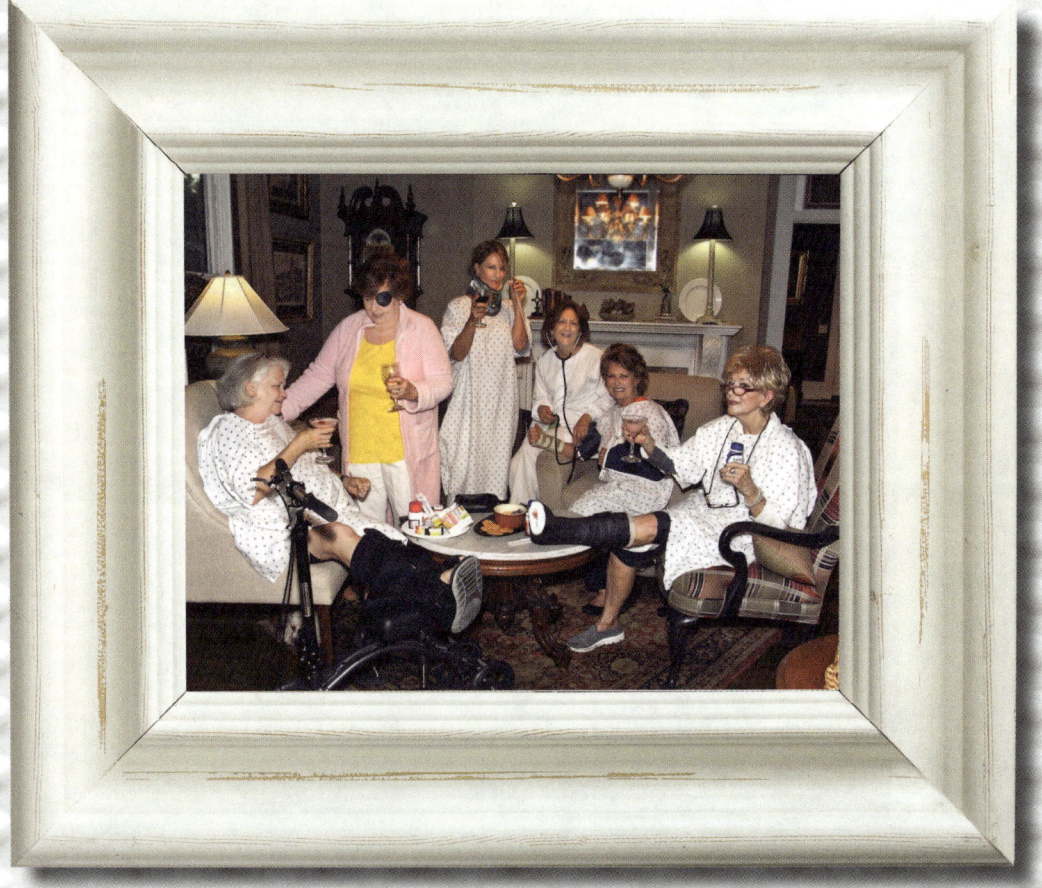

Stuff happens as we get older. Bones break, discs slip, and arthritis sets in. We find that getting together on a regular basis (with a lot of laughter) relieves any and all pain.

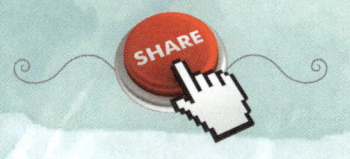

Hearing is the first thing to go for men

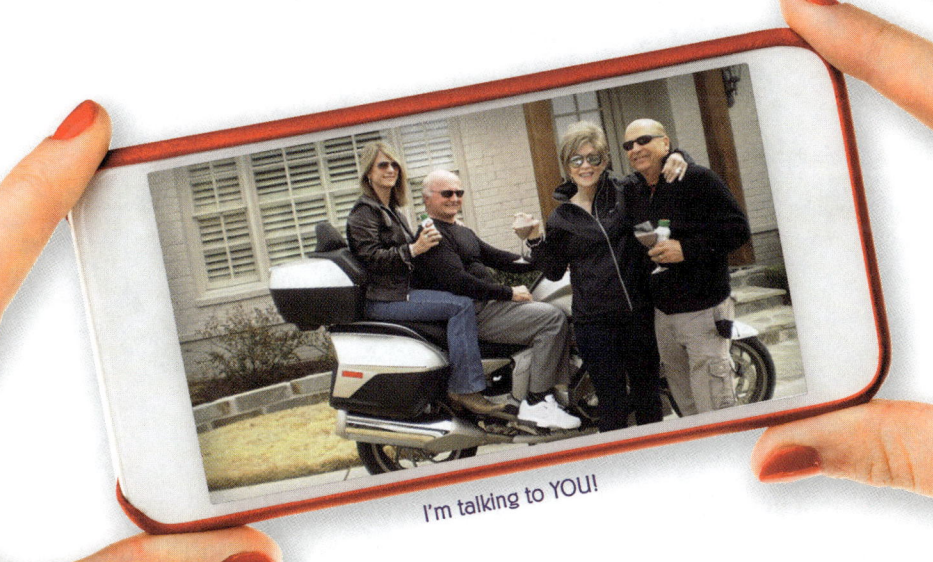

I'm talking to YOU!

This week, ten of my best high school buddies got together to officially launch plans for our fiftieth class reunion. Truth be told, it's probably more like our 150th reunion, because we get together at the drop of a hat. Nevertheless, we try to put on the dog at least every five years, and the fiftieth anniversary of our matriculation is cause to go all out and put on the dog and the pony!

We're even having it on the weekend of May 23, which is the very same weekend we received our diplomas all those decades ago. We intend to throw the greatest party ever to commemorate our enduring friendship. We even borrowed a line from the Bonnie Raitt hit tune *(Let's Give Them) Something To Talk About* as our theme.

> • • •
>
> "I don't want to brag or make anyone jealous … but I can still fit into the earrings I wore in high school."
>
> —Linda Barton Aultman, Class of 65

Scary, huh? What could a bunch of 67-year-olds possibly do to give anyone something to talk about? I don't know … maybe let the air out of our own tires, forcing us to stay out all night like we did after graduation. We could dance the night away just like fifty years ago, so long as the ambulance and a team of EMTs are on hand to resuscitate whomever needs resuscitating.

I expect we will play some games—spin the Geritol bottle,

do some Ensure shooters—anything but Kick the Can. At our age, that game will be banned for all future gatherings.

If this week's planning session is any indication of the widening gap between the male and female genders, I'm thinking we may need to hold separate reunions. Of the ten of us on the committee, only two are males. It became clear to me from the get-go that after a lifetime of tuning out the female voice, the male Eustachian tube has lost the ability to pick up vibrations from a woman. What do they hear when we speak? Crickets?

Case in point: I commented that we must go all out to make this our best reunion ever. Before I got it out of my mouth, the chairman cleared his voice and boomed, "Folks, this has got to be our best reunion ever." Okay, so his bad ear was on my side. Then the co-chairman, also a guy, hit his fist on the table and declared, "Listen up, kids! We've got to make this our best reunion ever." His bad ear was on both sides, apparently.

So with great fanfare and singleness of purpose, the girls discussed various ideas while the guys looked at us blankly. Suddenly, I recalled what it was like to be married. I'd seen that blank stare before.

While we planned, the guys mumbled to each other about who knows what—probably congratulating themselves on their award-winning depiction of the hearing-impaired (which I didn't believe for a moment). They also looked as though they were conjuring a bomb threat to force evacuation of the building.

We made one concrete decision: all classmates will be required to leave eyeglasses at home. We will all look better without magnification.

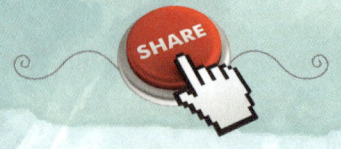

The crime of killing time

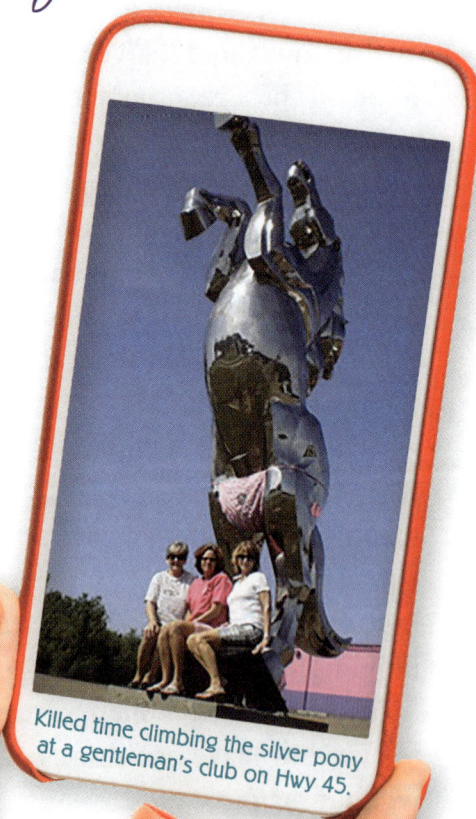

Killed time climbing the silver pony at a gentleman's club on Hwy 45.

If killing time were a crime, I should be labeled a serial murderer! I just spent twenty minutes looking for my reading glasses and finally found them hanging around my neck—on my new tortoise shell Peepers Eyeglass Holder chain.

And I've spent untold hours desperately looking for my cell phone while chatting with a friend on that very phone.

I became flummoxed by the thought of how much time I kill as I wait anxiously in front of the microwave. I had worked up an appetite while searching for my glasses and decided to thaw a piece of an Edward's Key Lime Pie (which requires only about fifteen seconds). It seemed like an eternity.

I watched the seconds tick away with one hand on the handle, practically foaming at the mouth in anticipation of the gooey citrus confection. It suddenly occurred to me that I was watching my life dwindle away with each tick of the microwave timer. Surely I could find a better way to spend it than by staring at a revolving microwave tray, right?

Time is a complex concept. Like it or not, we are all customers of the Bank of Time, according to Feng Shui enthusiasts I've been following on the internet. Every morning we are credited with 86,400 seconds. Every night The Bank charges off as a loss whatever time we have failed to invest in some good purpose. Now, it doesn't have to be productive, mind you. It can be totally selfish and pointless, but if you enjoy it, no "killing time" charges should be filed against you.

Such deep contemplation causes one to rethink a minute, which in turn triggers the beginning of a migraine. This is exactly why I don't think deeply very often.

An hour without any obligations can make us feel downright flush, but what do we do with it? These days it seems that most people stare at their cell phones as if expecting a genie to appear and grant them three wishes.

Your account in the Bank of Time carries no balance … well, except during the daytime hours, when you glance at your watch and realize how much time remains until you can call it a day.

The Bank of Time allows no overdrafts, though many of us live as though it does. My mother used to call it *burning the candle at both ends*, and I've done my share. Each day the same amount of time is deposited into your account, and each night you burn the remains of the day. If you fail to use the day's deposits on something that offers satisfaction or a contribution to humanity, you lose. There is no going back. No loans. No drawing against future deposits.

> • • •
>
> "Modern man thinks he loses something—time—when he does not do things quickly. Yet he does not know what to do with the time he gains, except kill it."
>
> —From *The Art of Loving* by Erich Fromm

I overheard an older gentleman comment the other day, "Sometimes I sits and think, and sometimes I just sits!" I can relate to that. Modern man thinks he loses time when he just sits. He is also inclined to do things as quickly as possible. But what do you do with the time you gain, except to kill it?

For me, standing in line is a brutal waste of time—as is getting caught in a traffic jam at rush hour when Highway

12 can look more like a used-car lot. I crank up the tunes and thank the good Lord that I'm stuck here and not in some place like New Jersey.

You're making withdrawals right this second and probably killing a little time if you're reading this insipid treatise. The days are long, but the years are short. Whatever we do—even if it bores us to tears—is a part of the fabric of our lives and worth appreciating with our senses fully alert. You never know when you might make a valuable memory.

Me? I'm going to do some creative loafing, which doesn't include use of the microwave or the remote control. It's called napping.

Liar, liar, pants on fire

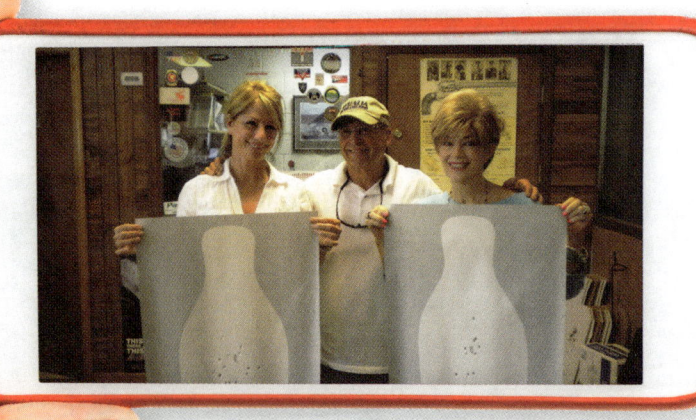

Marie, Heard, and I stretched the truth about our shooting skills.

A group of my "over 50" cronies were discussing our fascinating lives over coffee the other day. Two had just returned from a trip to Italy, one had been cross-country skiing in Wyoming, and the oldest of the group had just placed first in his age bracket in a half marathon.

Me? I had nothing. My big adventure was a trip out to Morgan Town to fill up a milk jug with spring water. Whoop-de-do. So I did something so reprehensible it's giving me nightmares: I casually mentioned that I was planning a trip to Albuquerque to participate in the Hot Air Balloon Races.

I have absolutely no idea where that came from. It just bubbled up like a giant hiccup and released itself before my mind had time to stop it. Such an adventure never has been, nor ever will be, on my bucket list. I cannot tolerate heights above about 24 inches, and the thought of sailing through the sky dangling from a balloon makes me catatonic.

However, members of my coffee klatch looked at me with new respect and began shooting questions about my big plans. I had no alternative except to answer with more tall tales and white lies (which were beginning to turn 50 shades of gray). I was very uncomfortable because my pants were on fire and my nose had grown into an elephant snout.

What causes otherwise sane individuals to resort to blatant subterfuge in order to make our lives sound more interesting than they really are? Now I have to go get some travel brochures and pretend to make plans to fly to New Mexico. All these lies will require another whopper—like a heart transplant or something equally critical—to give me a plausible reason to cancel the big balloon adventure that never was, and never will be.

See how that works? One small little white lie can create a monster that never goes away. After my heart transplant, they'll be asking if I will resume plans for the balloon races. I'm dead meat.

Consequently, I have begun to take inventory of the little white lies and tall tales I dispense so freely. How many of you have said, "I was just about to call you!" when someone calls you for the third time? You really weren't thinking about them, but you were going to get around to it eventually. Maybe.

How about, "You look great in those Bermuda shorts and knee socks!" while wondering if the guy has gone off his rocker.

"Officer, I was rushing home to let my dog out," I told the nice policeman who stopped me as I sped home from a basketball game the other night. Actually that one worked, but I got payback when greeted with a puddle at the back door.

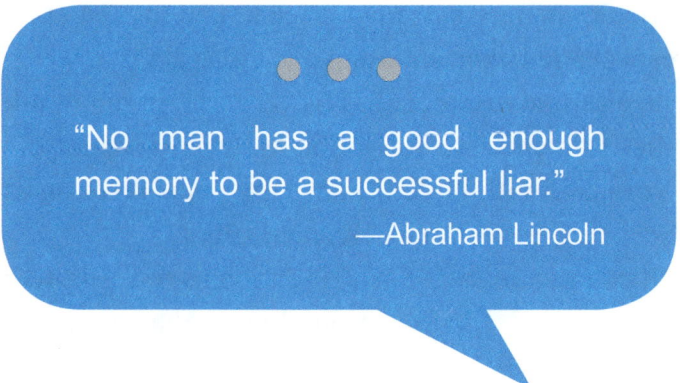

"No man has a good enough memory to be a successful liar."

—Abraham Lincoln

My policy has been that as long as we're not hurting others or breaking the law, a few little white lies can smooth over an abundance of sticky situations. It's when you begin to embellish the lie that you get yourself into trouble.

It occurs to me that I lie to myself about as much as anyone else. Every morning I begin the day promising to give up sugar in any form and eat a plant-based diet. By 3 p.m. I'm a drooling idiot lurking around the pastry bin at Walmart. Just one, I tell myself. By 6 p.m. I'm eating Nutella out of the jar with veggie chips—they're a vegetable, right?

I've decided to come clean and be brutally honest in all situations from now on, although I'll not be very popular. So don't ask my opinion about anything, or you might hear this: "Those jeans make you look fat and your homemade salad dressing tastes like motor oil."

Most of our innocent white lies serve as a kind of harmless social lubricant to make us more socially acceptable and likeable. Just be careful and don't cross the line as I did—and report a tale so tall only death itself can free you from the shame.

Of course, as the occasional teller of tall tales, my defense is that we should never muddy a perfectly good story with the facts.

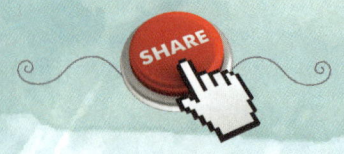

You're not who you were, only older

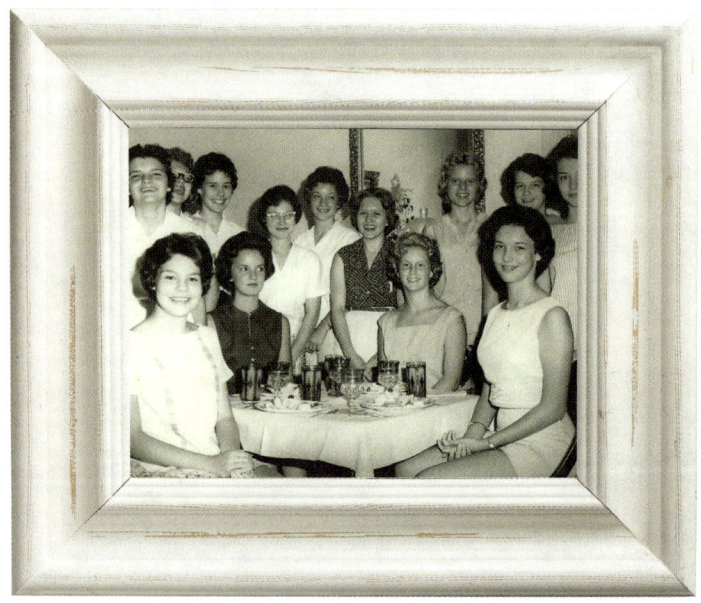

The way we were before we got the way we are

I woke up one morning after retiring for the third time from the nine-to-five world and going several rounds in the boxing ring with cancer. I had a horrifying thought that left me breathless—I didn't know who I was or what I was doing here since my life had shifted on its axis through the double whammy of age and illness.

All my life, I'd had clear roles to fill: wife, mother, daughter, chauffeur, editor, marketing director, housekeeper, chief cook and bottle washer … I could go on with an exhaustive list that makes me wonder where I found the time to get everything done. I'm sure there are many readers who could one-up me on my list!

> "We can't be afraid of change. You may feel very secure in the pond that you are in, but if you never venture out of it, you will never know that there is such a thing as an ocean, a sea. Holding onto something that is good for you now may be the very reason why you don't have something better."
>
> —Unknown

Now, at age 68, I'd been stripped of all those roles except *mother* and my children have busy lives of their own. Mothering them is little more than causing them angst that I will run off with some lothario or send my nest egg to a TV evangelist.

I had become a woman without a clear purpose; why was I put here besides keeping the doctors and drug companies in high cotton? What did I want to do with the rest of my life, other than sitting in my comfort zone and drooling in front of the television set?

Suddenly I had a flashback. I was a child splashing in the ocean without one single thought about my future. I was just getting to the stage where other people are trying to impose their expectations on me. (You can't possibly be a fire-woman. What would Grandma think?)

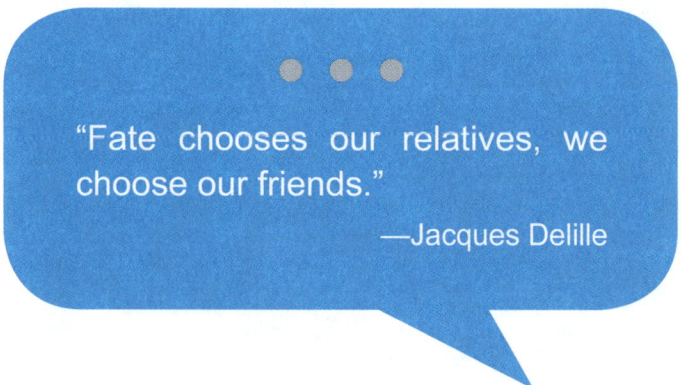

"Fate chooses our relatives, we choose our friends."

—Jacques Delille

What advice would the old geezer in me (who has been around the block a few times) give that innocent little child whose experience was limited only by her imagination? My first advice would be twofold: 1) Floss every day and 2) Go to Plumber School. I wish I had done both.

But then I began to get into the game. "You snot-nosed little twit, pull yourself together and stand up for yourself. You are shaping up to be a people-pleasing welcome mat and it will give you a lifetime of frustration. Don't do ANYTHING just to make someone else happy or earn their love and admiration."

I would tell her to follow her heart, no matter how unpopular that might be. I would tell her that money is a necessary evil, but it's not the main thing. I would tell her not to marry the first man who asks her after college graduation—even when she overheard her mother speculate that she would become an old maid. (That rarely turns out well, but you can get some fabulous children.)

I would tell her to never ever smoke a cigarette, because it would make her a slave and one day she would find herself standing outside her office building sucking on a cancer stick in the rain. (That's such a sad sight, and I don't see many men doing it. They must have a secret place.)

I would tell her to cultivate close friendships, which will carry her joyfully through the years and prove to be more supportive than family in some cases. We don't get to choose our families, but friends are ours for the picking ... and before you know it you're thinking of them as family.

So, what would you say to your little starry-eyed self? Or for that matter, what do you say to your cataract-producing, cloudy-eyed self? How do you take care of your body, mind, and your finances ... so they don't run out before you do?

You pull up your collar against the cold north wind and hope the coat you're wearing doesn't belong to someone else. You head into the unknown with faith that everything will be okay once you get your bearings. You figure out what it is you love doing, then go do it. You take some risks—and when they don't work, you try something else.

Summing up, you reinvent yourself when faced with stodginess—revising your schedule every day if necessary. And above all, you hope and pray you'll get your second wind and figure out at last what life's all about.

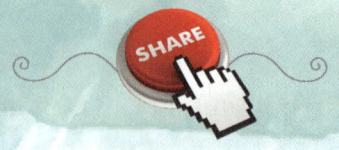

Bewildered by modern "slanguage"

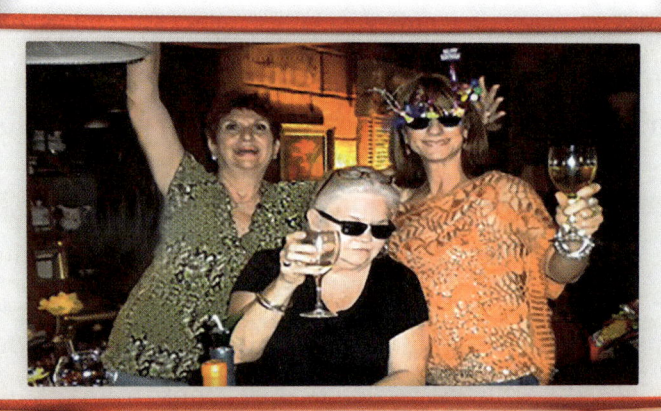

Ruthie, Linda, and Marie were cool
yesterday and hot today. Go figure.

I did it to my parents who did it to their parents. Now they're doing it to us, and I'm wondering if the King's English is already our second language.

Of course, I'm talking about slang. It swings, grooves,

rocks, and rules from generation to generation. Each has its own "slanguage" composed of puzzling pet phrases … which allow the youth in our culture to communicate while their elders remain clueless.

What was "23 skidoo" in the 1920s became "Let's roll" a century later. What was "jiving" in the 1930s became "groovin" in the 60s and "boss" in the 70s. What "burned you up" in the 50s will "frost" you in the new millennium.

> • • •
>
> No matter how much you spend on skin treatments or hair color to fight aging, it's what you say that gives you away.

Slang is probably no more puzzling today than it was two centuries ago when a thief was called a "smatter hauler" for stealing handkerchiefs. They couldn't steal credit cards, so they stole handkerchiefs, I suppose. The thief would be detained by the "crushers"—the 19th century equivalent of "cops."

Slang is a tribal thing, and I think my tribe (the over-50 crowd) is engaged in a hostile takeover. The rise of texting has complicated things even more. If you catch your grandchild texting "GPO," that's short for "grandparents over shoulder."

From flappers to rappers, slanguage has always been

around and it will reveal your age more quickly than you can say Botox. No matter how much you spend on skin treatments or hair color to fight aging, it's what you say that gives you away.

I was chatting with my twenty-something neighbor today and we were discussing work underway to install fiber optic cables along our street.

"Sweet," he remarked. "Well, I'll be a monkey's uncle," I said. He looked at me like I was a Twinkie at the health club. "Err, groovy," I corrected myself. He said nothing, but I saw the brief eye roll. When did I cross the Grand Canyon from hip young career woman to 1934 Studebaker?

What we once called a newcomer would soon be shortened by email to "newbie" and more recently to just plan noob. Noob is used to describe someone from the dark ages—like a parent. A simple phrase like "None of your business" has been replaced by "Nunya." To say "Good job" on television has become a "shout-out" and everyone's doing it from the president to Sponge Bob Square Pants.

And you haven't lived until you've been "dissed" by someone. Apparently getting dissed is not a good thing and involves being the butt of someone's joke. I heard the verb used five times today and had to run and look it up to discover that it's a modern form of disrespect.

Okay. I think I've got it. I've been practicing: "You dissin' me, noob?" I'm just not sure when to use it.

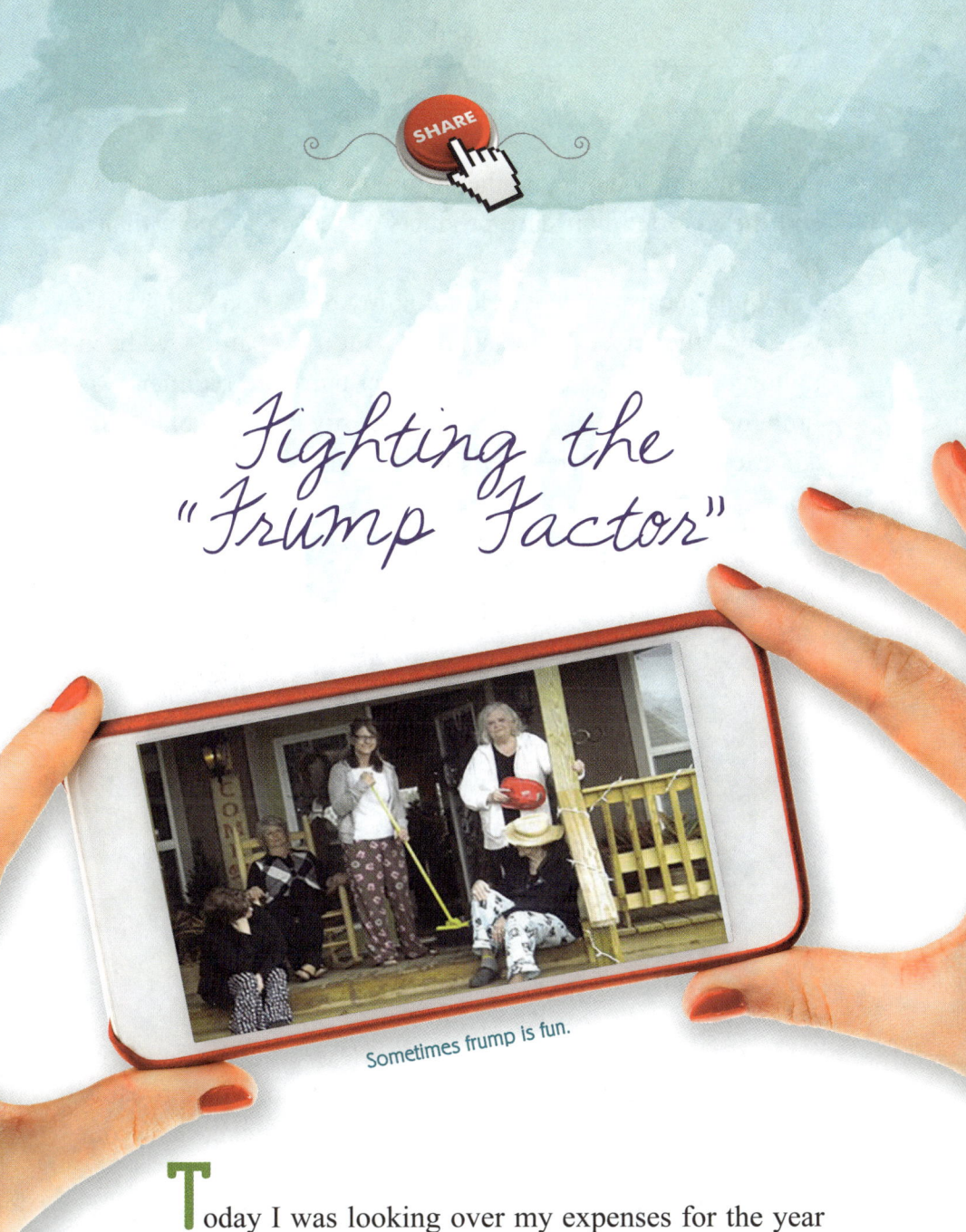

Fighting the "Frump Factor"

Sometimes frump is fun.

Today I was looking over my expenses for the year and was flabbergasted to see what I've spent on my hair in the past twelve months. It was obscene. I could have financed a small country, yet the bad hair days still outnumber the good about 20 to 1.

The monthly hair cuts, the bi-monthly gray-zapping color, and the assorted hair care products added up to more than I spend on food.

I know most people would think my obsession with hair is way over the top and I'm ashamed. But it's a battle I've been fighting since I was twelve, when my hair care regimen was limited to a bit of sugar water to paste my bangs in place and a bottle of Prell which lasted an entire year.

> ● ● ●
>
> "If you're having a bad hair day, try not to complain—there are a lot of folks out there with cancer who would kill just to have hair at all."
>
> —Norma Atkins, who fought like a soldier to help take care of her friend Frances Hill, who died of cancer this spring

Does anyone remember Prell? If you do, you probably shouldn't admit it, because it will date you quicker than your laugh lines.

I'm still trying to find an escape for the "frump slump" which has been flirting with me for months. So I looked around at my friends who seem to have developed an immunity to this malady.

My friend Janie was the first to come to mind. She enters a room looking like a million bucks with bouncy modern hair and so put together—while I'm crawling around on the floor trying to retrieve a shoulder pad that fell out when I was trying to smooth out my Spanx. Bummer. (I'm probably the only female on the planet who still wears shoulder pads—even with a T-shirt. I think that little boost gives me an athletic look … like I've been working out in the gym.)

One day I sucked up my pride and asked Janie how she got her hair to behave so beautifully. I'm still trying to recreate that "big hair" look with two-thirds less hair, which comes with aging in my family.

She gave me a list of what I needed to get smoking hot (or at least lukewarm) hair. I rushed out and grabbed it all. I bought #12 Rough Play Paste, Big Sexy Powder Play, Smoking Bedhead Gel and What a Tease Backcomb in a Bottle. It all sounded like the ingredients for a cheap porn flick.

I washed my hair and applied all the products as directed and, for once in my life, I had big beautiful hair. At church the following Sunday no one would sit behind me because they couldn't see the pastor over my hair. It was a glorious moment.

It was hard separating my hair from the pillow each morning, but I was one happy girl. Of course, now that I held the secret, the unexpected occurred. Cancer set in, and treatment swept all the big hair away. But the lesson I learned is that hair really isn't all that important in the scheme of things.

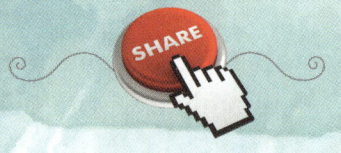

Who shrunk my groceries?

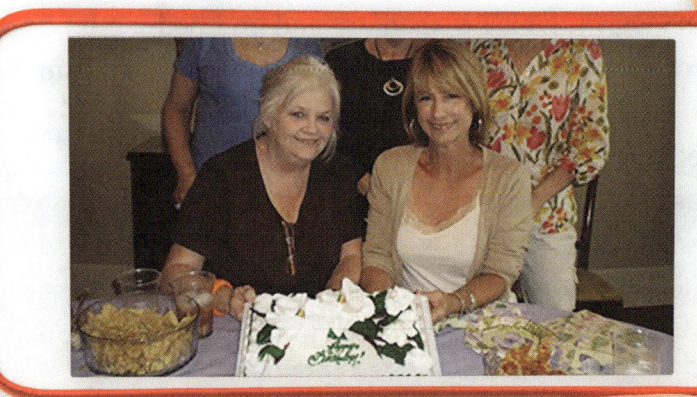

Ironically, birthday cakes are getting bigger to accommodate more candles.

Ironically, as Americans grow bigger, the food companies are shrinking the packages we place in our grocery carts each week. Go figure. This situation has left cooks all over the country scratching their heads while trying to figure out how to translate Grandmother's traditional recipes using the scaled-down ingredients.

If anyone deserves the Naughty Award this year, it's the big corporate food packers who have gotten together and tried to fool shoppers by shaving the packaging ever so slightly in some cases, and ever so grandly in others.

What? They think we won't notice that Kraft American cheese went from 24 slices to 22? That Tropicana orange juice went south by 7.8 percent, and Haagen Dazs ice cream shrunk by 12.5 percent? Frankly, I didn't notice until someone pointed out that cake mixes, the basis of so many wonderful confections, have been tampered with.

The typical 18.25-ounce box of cake mix has mysteriously lost a few ounces. This little *sleight of hand* is likely responsible for culinary failures taking place across the country. That's my excuse!

Has anyone else experienced the confusion surrounding treasured family recipes based on the size of cans and mixes dating to the 1930s (when convenience packaging first appeared on the general store shelves)?

My recipe for Blueberry/Pineapple Cobbler is a good example of the corporate plot to destroy our beloved traditions. The recipe calls for one box of yellow cake mix, one can of blueberry pie filling, one large can of slivered pineapple, a stick and a half of butter, and a cup of nuts. The beauty of this scrumptious cobbler is that it takes one pan and a modicum of dexterity to open the can. To make the recipe work this year, I will have to compute and adjust all the other ingredients to accommodate the smaller cake mix. My math is just not that good.

I'm pretty furious about this, and I called the corporate office of Pillsbury to register my disappointment. They put me on hold and I had to listen to elevator music until I went into a coma. I'm sure there are people everywhere puzzled by this blatant subterfuge. Not only has the cost of the cans and mixes increased, we are getting less to boot. I guess they figure that if exorbitant gasoline prices haven't stopped us from driving, a half cup shaved off our cake mixes won't stop us from baking.

> • • •
>
> "Consumers are discovering more air in their bag of chips, fewer sheets of paper towels on the roll, thinner garbage bags and even smaller squares of toilet paper."
>
> —CNN Money

Just recently, Kimberly-Clark announced that Kleenex would have 13 percent fewer sheets, but would make their tissues 15 percent "bulkier" by adding more fiber. What kind of society has healthier tissues than human beings (who incorporate way too little fiber in their diets)? And even if the size of my peanut butter jar looks the same, it now sports an inward dimple on the bottom which effectively reduces the amount of product in the jar. The wine producers were the first to discover that one. I've also noticed that a bag of potato chips is mostly air these days.

Next, I expect our sticks of butter to be reduced in size, which will destroy the remainder of the recipes in my file box. The only thing we can depend on is the size of a nut, and thank goodness corporate America had nothing to do with that.

How to become a shut-in

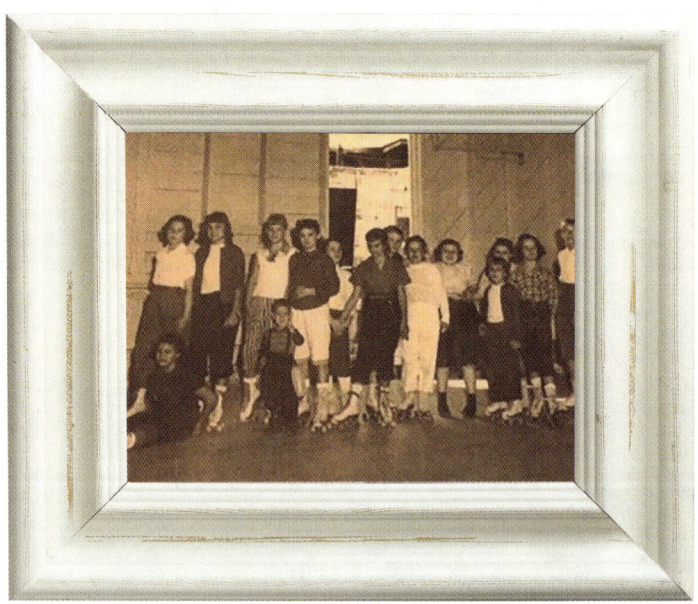

In our youth, TV was an activity of last resort, and skating parties were just invented

I am in the midst of the worst break-up of my life and I'm working on recovery with every tool at my disposal.

It all began when my well-intentioned children installed

more electronic "whatchamathingies" on my television sets. In addition to Netflix, I have something called Sling and Ikono which provide unlimited streaming of every series or movie ever produced.

But Netflix is my drug of choice and apparently I'm not alone. The phenomenon known as "binge-watching" Netflix has spread across the globe as network TV continues to feature mindless programming, and Netflix cranks out fascinating programs at the speed of light. The service provides nonstop exposure to what we once called Soaps, but with much better characters and story lines (and a whole lot racier).

You can keep watching as long as you are there and awake to punch the button when your screen sends up the prompt ARE YOU STILL WATCHING? Can you believe your TV can carry on a conversation with you these days? Since there are no commercial breaks, you have exactly 17 seconds between episodes to get up and do a push-up (which is the sum total of my exercise program).

Netflix streaming increased 350 percent from 2013-2015. Users watched a mind-boggling *seven billion* hours of Netflix in three months. I can account for several hundred, and I haven't left the house except to replenish my stash of micro-wave popcorn and Lean Cuisines.

And get this, my credit card company sent me a warning that Netflix has become a national health hazard. I guess they noticed that I'm not spending any money or charging anything on the card except for the monthly Netflix fee—a measly $8.55 a month. Gosh, if this continues, it could destroy the already fragile economy.

But it gets worse. Research from the *Journal of the American Heart Association* shows that users who view more than three hours of television per day are more at risk for heart disease, stroke, and even cancer. Three hours? That's only an appetizer for me.

My eyes are itchy and swollen, and my muscles have begun to atrophy. Of course, my emotions are all over the place depending on whether I'm watching a comedy or a tragedy. I call it Nexapause; menopause is a piece of cake by comparison.

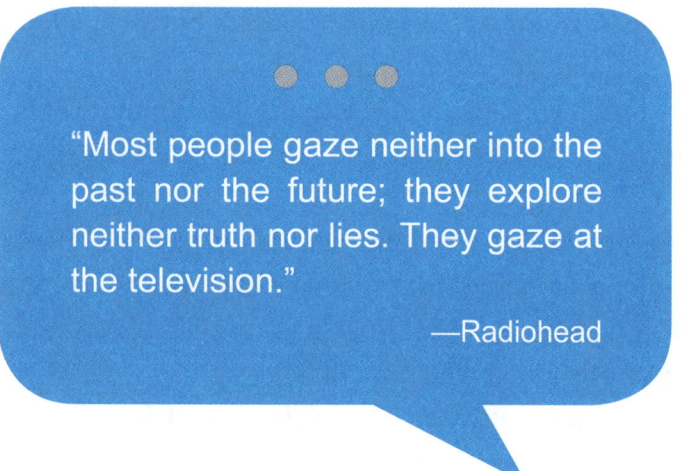

"Most people gaze neither into the past nor the future; they explore neither truth nor lies. They gaze at the television."

—Radiohead

I'm pretty sure nobody on their death bed ever wished they'd spent more time watching Netflix. After watching for almost a solid month and not getting dressed or answering the phone, I made up my mind that such behavior must come to an abrupt halt.

My voluntary shut-in status demanded radical measures to break the habit. So at an advanced age and with a bad Netflix hangover, I came out of retirement and took a job as temporary editor of my local newspaper. After seven years of retirement from the nine-to-five workaday world, I tore myself away from the house and television and made an effort to become a productive citizen again.

My advice is this: If you have reached a certain age when staying home and lounging around in your PJs seems preferable to exciting social events and you don't yet have Netflix, don't get it. And if you do subscribe, you better have a part-time job or an absorbing hobby to pry you away most hours of the day.

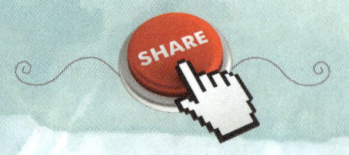

Got everything done— died anyway

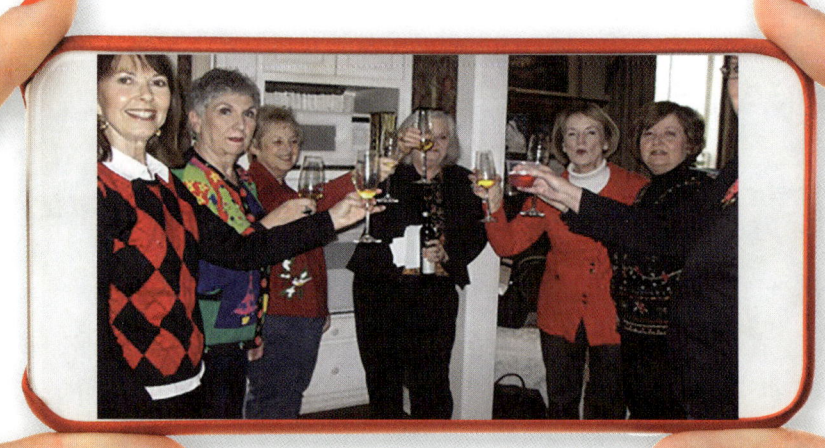

Our to-do list always includes celebration.

It came to me suddenly, like a bolt of lightning from the sky. I have begun taking my daily to-do list to the extreme.

You know you've crossed that line when the number one item on your list is DO THE TO-DO LIST. That way I can accomplish one thing, even if it's only the making of the list.

The second warning sign is when you do something on a whim and go back and add it to the list just so you can check it off. I do both of these things on a regular basis, and now I learn that such behavior may be an early sign of obsessive compulsive disorder (OCD).

Oh great. I can add another malady to my already malady-filled life.

I've been making lists since I learned how to write in first grade. My first entry was, "Write letter to Mr. Santa Claus," and when he actually came down the chimney and delivered my most coveted toys, my fate was sealed. I would become a loyal list-maker for the rest of my life in hopes that some cosmic Santa would make all my plans miraculously happen.

So I begin each day with a list of chores, goals, and needs. It's no big deal if the item doesn't get checked; I move it forward until I'm sick of looking at it. After a couple of weeks it drops off into a black hole, never to be seen again. That's why a new section of fencing out back will never get painted. I pretend I'm waiting for the wood to cure, but to tell the truth I hate painting, especially the prep and necessary clean-up.

My headstone should read: "Got everything done—died anyway." I try to repeat that sentence in my head throughout the day to put it all into perspective.

Frankly, the to-do list has become a crutch. It's an anchor in the storm of life when I become overwhelmed by all that needs doing. Making the list means I don't have to actually deal with it until the list is complete. Sometimes it can take an hour or more … when I could be actually doing the chore!

Another warning sign that list-making has run amok is when you search all over town for just the right notebook to contain the list, and of course you need the perfect pen to perform the perfect ritual. When that pen goes missing, I turn the house upside down to find it before I can complete the list. By this time, the list has become an evil form of procrastination.

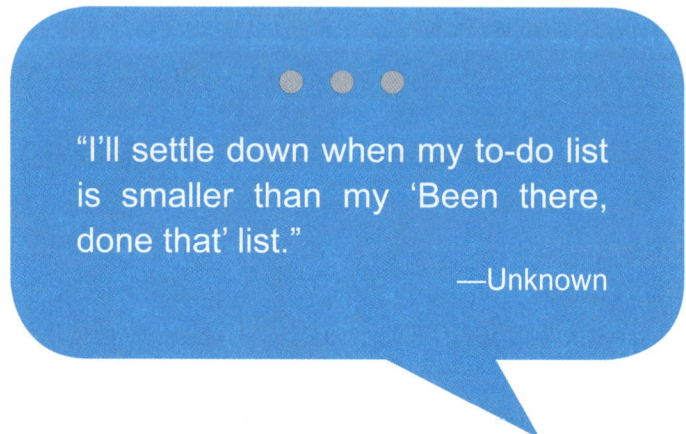

"I'll settle down when my to-do list is smaller than my 'Been there, done that' list."

—Unknown

I suspect the real reason some people make detailed lists is a desperate attempt to gain some sense of control in a world which is spinning seriously out of control. We are pulled in so many directions by our toys (cell phones, emails, and Facial Book; I call it Facial Book just to tick it off). Tekkie toys interrupt our focus and spawn new items on the to-do list.

Sometimes I feel like the little steel ball in a pinball machine. Someone pulls the trigger and I go bouncing off everything in sight; then, as I head into the home stretch, a little flipper pops up and sends me back out into the minefield.

This week I experimented with going *without* my list for one day, just to see if I could live without it. I never got dressed or ventured outside the house, although I must say it was a delightful day and I piddled and puttered with no real direction. Ironically, it turned out to be my most productive day in months. Seems if I don't HAVE to do something, I'm more likely to do it.

Starting now, I'm limiting my to-do list to three things that cannot wait another day without rendering myself homeless, malnourished, or cited for loitering. I'm calling it the "Ta Da" list, and it includes only those things which—when done—will give me the feeling I have conquered the world. That means I will do 1) one hard thing I've been pushing forward, 2) one thing to help someone beside myself, and 3) one thing that makes my heart sing and puts me in the "zone," where I lose all track of time.

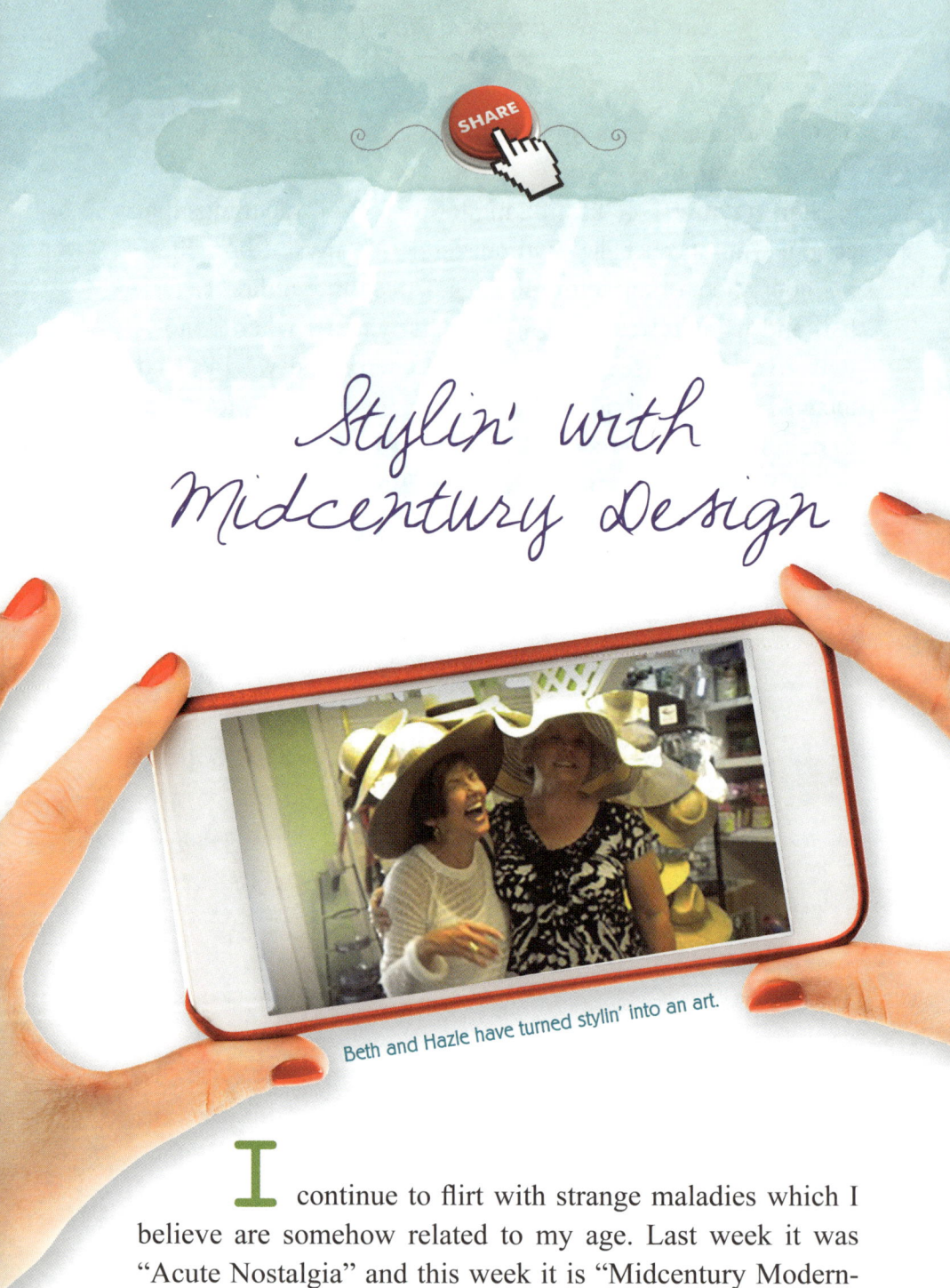

Stylin' with Midcentury Design

Beth and Hazle have turned stylin' into an art.

I continue to flirt with strange maladies which I believe are somehow related to my age. Last week it was "Acute Nostalgia" and this week it is "Midcentury Modern-itus." I'm pretty sure the latter could be costly. What gives?

Acute Nostalgia is a chronic condition that is easily relieved by sitting around remembering the good ole days, while Midcentury Modernitus involves a complete change in personal style—a tragedy for someone who has always loved nineteenth century collectibles and anything over the age of 100.

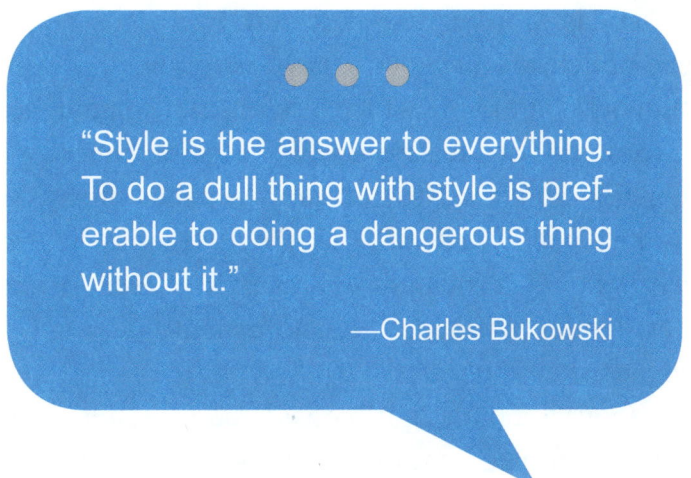

"Style is the answer to everything. To do a dull thing with style is preferable to doing a dangerous thing without it."

—Charles Bukowski

I suspect the two maladies are closely related and generally afflict people born between the years of 1946 and 1964. The renewed interest in 50s and 60s decor elicits memories from happy times for most Boomers. More likely it's because I just watched seven seasons of *Mad Men* (which is set in the 60s) and am completely enamored with Don Draper, who plays the dual role of protagonist and antagonist. He has a very cool wardrobe and even cooler Midcentury office furniture.

Okay, so since the dawn of human civilization, we have looked to the past for inspiration. But that doesn't explain an obsession with Midcentury Modern, arguably the tackiest period in recent history.

Suddenly, the dark, heavy antiques I've collected since my

twenties seem depressive and I'm looking for cleaner lines and less clutter. Something in my brain has shifted and bucket seats, tulip tables, and drum lamps are looking good to me. I gave away the monster-sized old desk in my home office last week and ordered a 60s reproduction of the tulip table—white, round, with a pedestal base. I even found a faux bear rug at Tuesday Morning to go under it.

Since giving up my desk, I have no drawers in which to stuff things I don't know where else to put. I'm going to have to buy (or build) bookcases in which to stash paperwork and memorabilia from the 50s, like my vintage Johnny Mathis albums and cookbooks such as the Elvis classic *Are You Hungry Tonight?* It includes his mama's recipes for mashed potatoes, lemon meringue pie, and peanut butter and 'nana sandwiches.

Until about a month ago I considered this style devoid of personality. I suspect that its revival is a form of rebellion—a desire for something simpler, probably in response to our fast-paced, multitasking, over-informed, frantic, fractured, Ethernet-driven lives.

Furniture and home decor that reflect an idealized vision of one's early days can also provide comfort and a sense of connection and security in uncertain times.

I'm not going whole hog, mind you. Just a touch here, maybe a disco ball in my dining room (and a clothesline in my garden). That kind of thing. Right now I'm feeling the need to mix up a Jell-O salad and watch a couple of episodes of *Perry Mason*. Ah, the good ole days. I feel at home at again.

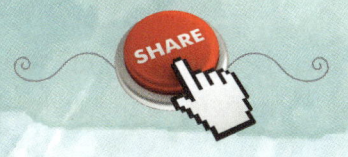

Sleepless in Starkville

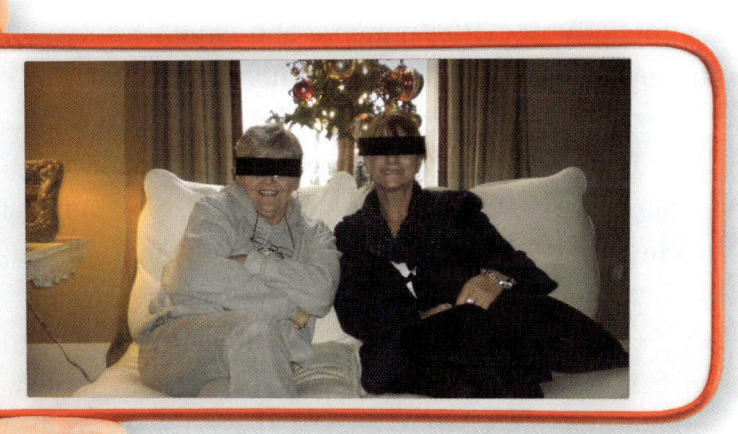

Our special glasses allow us to nap and no one knows.

Sleep has never been my strong suit and a little age has made it worse. Nightly tossing and turning with random thoughts churning through my head are more my style, and many mornings I get out of bed half past dead.

Four hours of sleep is a good night, and I've been known to operate heavy machinery (like the dishwasher and washing machine) on less than two. It's as if the world might be overrun by some encroaching calamity which my wakefulness is somehow fending off.

Consequently, I live in a perpetual state of jet lag, although I haven't left the ground since I jetted to Austin in 2007. Apparently I'm not alone in my chronic state of sleep deprivation. Every magazine I pick up features an article on the importance of sleep and how to get more without taking prescription medication. I've flatly refused to resort to sleeping pills because I read they can cause sleepwalking, eating, and driving in your sleep. With my luck I'd probably drive over to McDonald's each night for a quarter pounder and large fries, without ever knowing why I can no longer zip my jeans.

I've tried all the suggestions, like using blackout curtains and no caffeine after noon. I've tried melatonin, tryptophan, St. John's wort, chamomile, kava kava, and antihistamines. No amount of Celestial Bedtime tea helps (and it results in a lot of late-night trips to the bathroom).

A friend swears she has found blessed relief from sleep deprivation and other ailments by wearing something called a hematite ring. It's a sort of crystal that purportedly absorbs all your negative energy, allowing you to relax and sleep like a baby. It sounded like a bunch of hooey to me, but I read up on it and sure enough, one report claims the stone can absorb so much negativity they explode. To test the report, I've ordered rings for each hand. Stay tuned.

Admittedly, my acute insomnia is due in part to my strange bedfellows: a fuzzy poodle desperately in need of a shower, a bulldog named Rebel who snores like a freight train, and now a stray cat named Cat who vibrates the bed with her purring. All this is compounded by intermittent hissing and growling which I think may be coming from me. Oh, and did I mention I leave the television on all night? It's a habit I can't seem to break because some television shows are so lame they lull me to sleep.

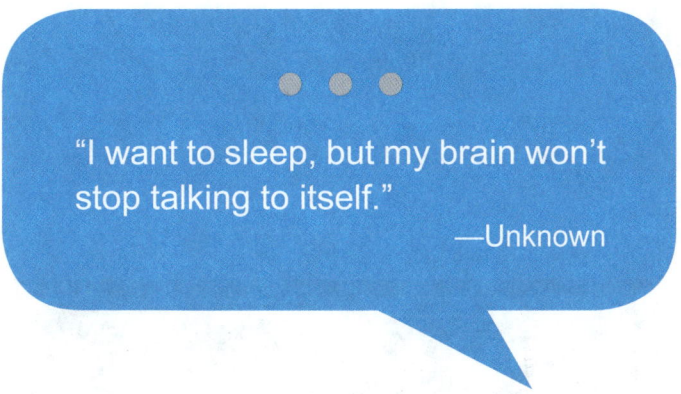

"I want to sleep, but my brain won't stop talking to itself."
—Unknown

Insomniacs in the Middle Ages were instructed to drink a potion made from the gall bladder of a castrated boar. I checked with the Piggly Wiggly, but they were flat out of boar. Fried lettuce is a French folk remedy, while chewing on sea slug entrails is a Japanese folk solution. Someone suggested eating a raw onion before bedtime, but it just made me cry myself to sleep.

The irony is that I get seriously drowsy in church or when I'm driving to some distant location alone. Go figure.

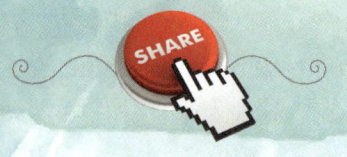

Sun rises on dark night of the soul

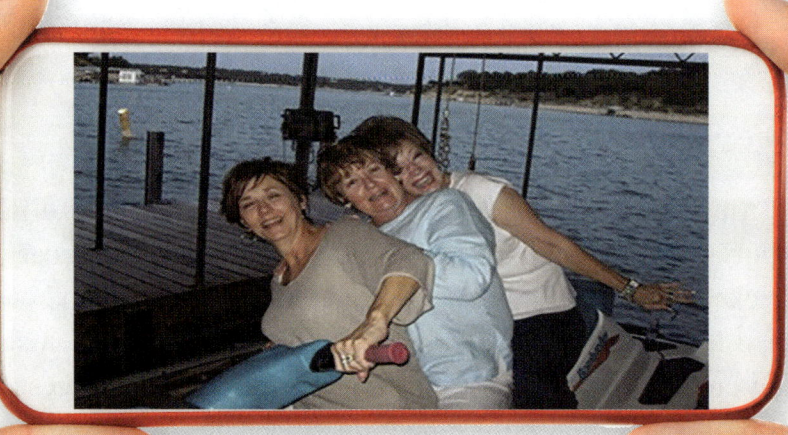

The morning after the dark night of the soul is pure fun.

"It was a dark and stormy night …" Don't most bad mysteries begin with those melodramatic and kitschy words? They have become so widely recognized that even Carl Schulz depicted Snoopy on the roof of his doghouse typing the phrase.

I recently experienced such a night, only it was complicated by what one sixteenth century author coined "the dark night of the soul." Such a personal downer can occur when less than happy circumstances stack up all at one time and you collapse under the weight of it all.

Most folks can handle one or two disasters at a time, but occasionally the planets line up in such a way that every dark thought you've ever had comes at you with the speed of an eighteen-wheeler going 100 miles an hour. I think they once called it a nervous breakdown. We are probably far too sophisticated for that in today's world.

My dark night came recently after losing my best friend of eighteen years, which dredged up every bad thing that has ever happened. I have a nasty tendency to sweep every mildly unpleasant thing under the rug. I'm a great rug sweeper because it's so much easier than dealing with the problems outright. I have become mentally adept at ignoring the two-ton elephant in the middle of the room until I cannot find a place to sit.

My dark night was brought on by many things: putting off things that needed doing three years ago; facing the ferocious acceleration of time that comes with the late middle ages; a bad chest cold I chose to ignore until it turned into the flu; a cancer diagnosis. Bummer. Watching nine seasons of *Brothers & Sisters*, a thinly-disguised prime-time soap opera on Netflix, didn't help.

I found myself turning down party invitations and not getting dressed so I could participate in daily marathons of this mind-numbing, albeit highly entertaining show. When Rob Lowe was killed off in one of the last episodes, I began wearing black and sent flowers to myself.

After the darkness descended, I rushed to my home library (an eight-foot-long bookcase tucked into a hallway) and grabbed my copy of *The Dark Night of the Soul*, which was penned in the sixteenth century by a Carmelite monk. It's not an easy read, but the rewards are many and equivalent to at least thirty sessions with a therapist. At $3.15 on Amazon, it was the bargain of all bargains.

Here's my favorite quote about those dark times, which was passed along to me by Keith Mooney of West Point, Mississippi:

● ● ●

"When you come to the edge of all the light you have and take the first step into the darkness of the unknown, you must believe one of two things will happen: You will be given something solid to stand upon or you will be taught how to fly."

—Unknown

St. John of the Cross authored this magnificent literary work as a guide on how to win the war between the soul (our higher selves) and the ego (the part of us which should be locked in the basement). If we follow St. John's recommendations, the ego will suffer a coronary and be put out of commission for an extended period of time—or until we begin sweeping stuff under the rug again.

In a nutshell, the monk's prescription is to lean into the darkness and experience the full consequences of all our sorrows and imperfections. All this soul-searching leads us back to God. And like magic, we stop deflecting the love and beauty that is all around us. That mysterious weather in our heads clears up and the sun rises again in glorious Technicolor.

Over the years I've observed that the greatest challenges can sometimes bring the greatest blessings. Oh, and one more thing to remember: The things you put out in the world— joyful or hateful—will always come back to bless you or haunt you. Your choice.

I guess you could call *The Dark Night of the Soul* the ultimate expression of spring cleaning. After the winter from hell which occurred in Mississippi in 2014-15, I'm ready for some spring cleaning. Today I'm sweeping up all the messes, but they are going to the curb, NOT under the rug. Besides, I'm reminded that there so many other exciting things going on in the world. After all, today is Senior Citizen Day at Walgreens ...

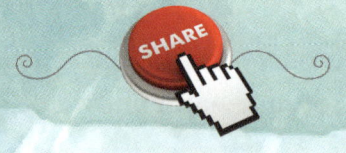

Declutter so you can reclutter

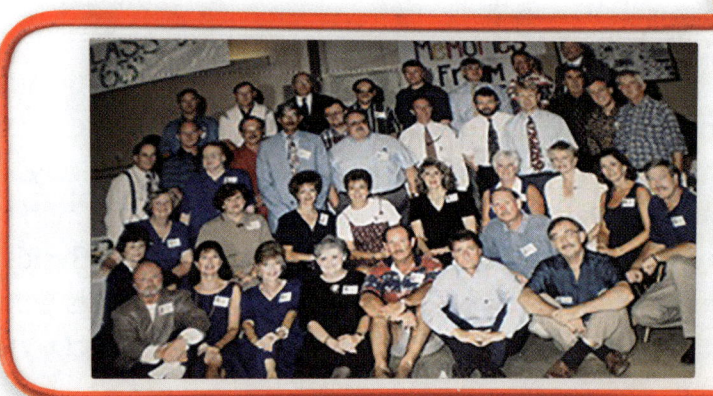

The one thing you never have too much of is old friends.

"The barn burned down, now I can see the moon." I don't remember where I heard that statement, but it sums up my need to declutter periodically.

For 33 consecutive days the number one item on my daily

120

To-Do list has been "spend twenty minutes decluttering my house." I sit at the computer for hours googling decluttering tips, but I haven't actually gotten around to taking any action.

In fact, it took me a half hour to find the computer under a mountain of junk that I don't know where to file. I was determined to get organized in 2015 and here it is July and I haven't even begun.

Meanwhile, clutter and doodads I don't even recognize are building to the point I may have to buy a bigger home. I'm not a hoarder, mind you. I'm just a collector.

It has come to my attention that perhaps I'm going about it all wrong. Home organization blogger Karen Clemons hit me squarely between the eyes with her tongue-in-cheek list of suggestions on how to INCREASE our clutter. Here are a few of her simple steps (along with a few of my own) outlining how to get that homey, *lived-in* look. I guess you could call me a maximalist rather than a minimalist, which is so chic these days. (Chic doesn't live here any more—in fact it never has.)

1. Always bring home the freebies—the booklets at museums, the soaps at the hotel, the pens at the bank. Never use them. But just bring them home. Last year I finally cleaned out the junk drawer so they could all be crammed in there.

2. Hang onto the heirlooms that you don't really like and display them in the center of your living room just because they belonged to someone you knew. Never, ever have any open spaces on your tables or walls. Place some decorative accent item on every square inch. That way the dust won't show.

3. Always have two of everything. It's useful to have a second can opener in case the first one breaks when you're opening a can of tuna.

4. Save crayon stubs because you might make them into candles one day.

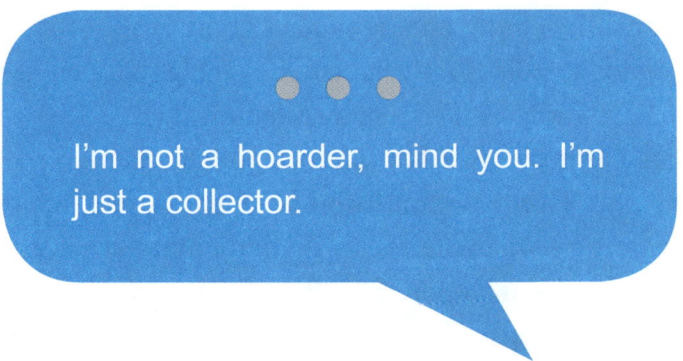

I'm not a hoarder, mind you. I'm just a collector.

5. Keep every greeting card and note you've ever received. And not just the romantic ones from your husband or boyfriend, but also the kid you babysat in 1965.

6. Keep everything. Keep a box of really short strings. Label it "Strings too short to use."

7. Always clean and store every spaghetti jar, soup can, Cool Whip container, paper towel roll, or toilet paper roll for some future but as-yet-undetermined use.

8. Never donate or toss clothes that have magically shrunk while hanging in the closet, because you just KNOW you're going to fit into those stone-washed, size four jeans again one day.

9. Don't discard anything that could be worth something someday. It is highly unlikely that thousands of others are saving the same items, thus increasing future value. How else would anything grow old enough to be an antique? You'll be doing a valuable public service by saving that thingamadoochie for future generations.

10. But there's always this: You may acquire so much clutter it won't matter so much if the house burns down.

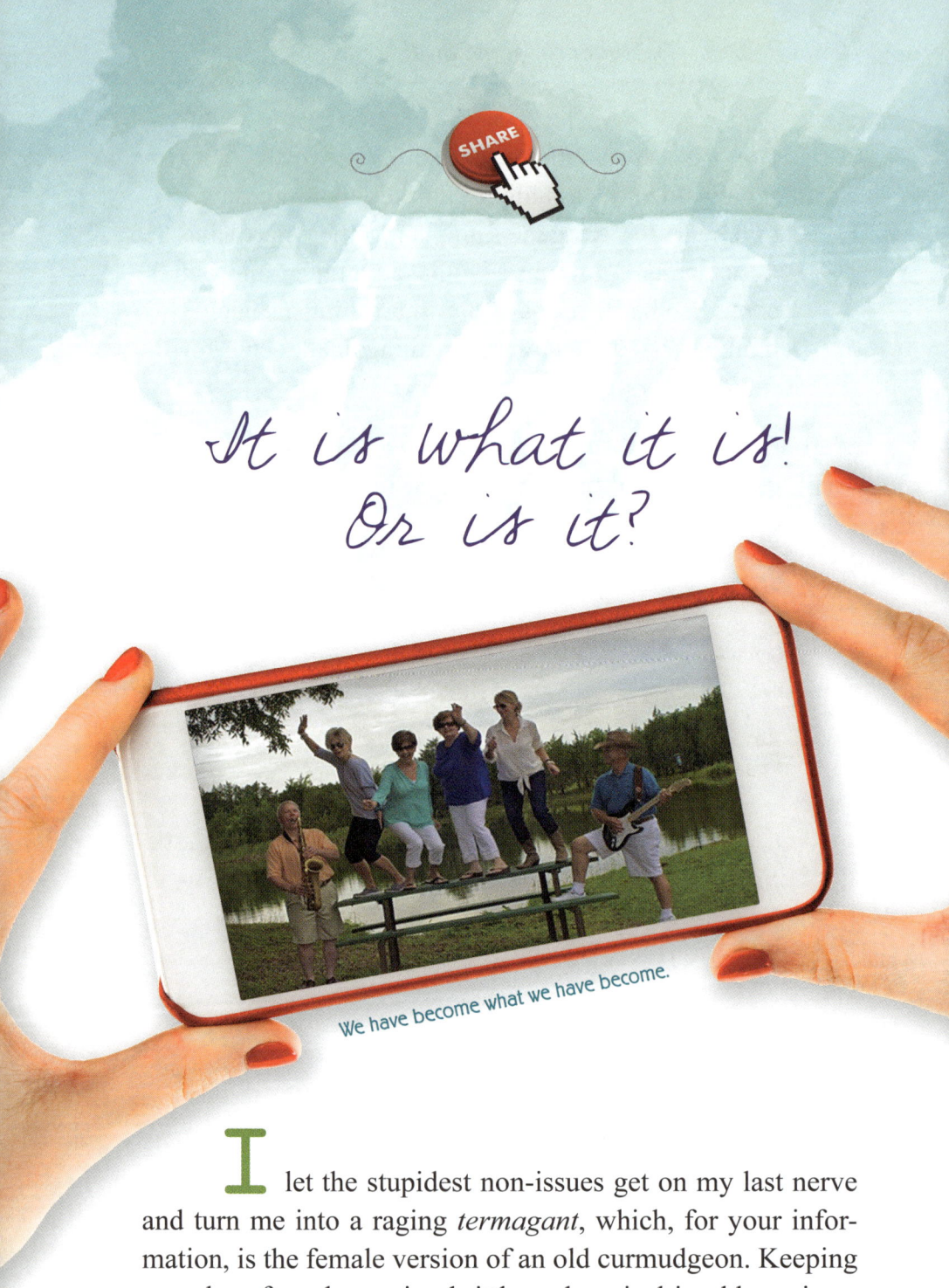

It is what it is! Or is it?

We have become what we have become.

I let the stupidest non-issues get on my last nerve and turn me into a raging *termagant*, which, for your information, is the female version of an old curmudgeon. Keeping ourselves from becoming brittle and cynical in old age is an ongoing challenge.

Remember that word (termagant) because if you're female you're probably carrying the gene. The condition begins to present itself with advancing age and loss of the inhibitions which once kept us civil and gave us the reputation as "sweet young thangs." The aging beauty can turn into the beast about the time she notices her neck is growing CREEPY. But hey, it is what it is, right? Wrong!

This phrase makes me bristle every time I hear it. It is popular with today's sports figures and politicians because, like all clichés, it helps them avoid speaking about the real issues.

In a recent *Time* Magazine survey, "It is what it is" ranked right up there with "Just Sayin'" and "Whatever" as the most annoying contemporary expressions, and which should pass immediately into oblivion.

It is what it is. My mental panty hose get in a wad every time I hear that ridiculous, worn-out, pseudo-intellectual statement. Well, *of course* it is what it is, Einstein! How could it be what it's not? The first time I overheard someone say, "It is what it is," I was almost relieved. Then I thought it through and realized the phrase excuses all sorts of bad behavior and conditions which could be remedied.

I tested the premise in my own life. My thighs are fine, thank you very much. Go ahead and pass me a chocolate-covered donut—no, make that the whole bag, because there's nothing I can do about my thighs or anything else in this ole world. It is what it is, and what will be will be. (Do they make sweat pants in size 75? Because that's what I'll be needing very soon.)

See what I mean? *It is what it is* represents the ultimate

cop-out, hinting there's not one thing in the world you can do anything about at all, so just go ahead and wallow in the messes of your life. Well, not *yours* specifically. I'm thinking of our collective messes, like litter on the highways and cruelty to animals. Hey, no problem, it is what it is. I think not, and the termagant lurking in my brain is about to get riled up all over again.

> It is what it is represents the ultimate cop-out, hinting there's not one thing in the world you can do anything about at all, so just go ahead and wallow in the messes of your life.

I'm about to ram the rear of a vehicle because the driver is stopped at a green light texting on his cell phone while traffic is backed up to the moon. BAM! He hops out of his car screaming at me and I reply blithely, "Settle down, junior, it is what it is." See how society could disintegrate into a million pieces if we lived by those five words?

So, please, America. Let's adopt some new expressions. My personal favorite is "Alrighty, then," which means whatever you want it to mean. "Alrighty then, sweetie! You are forgiven!" I equate it with "Don't sweat the small stuff; it is water under the bridge; and it will all come out in the wash!" Alrighty then, you termagants and curmudgeons. Wear your wrinkles proudly and don't hide those Ace bandages on your arthritic knees. That's the one time you're allowed to say "They are what they are."

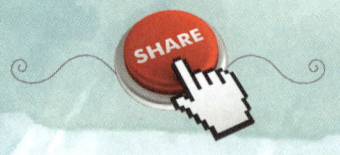

Invasion of the Belligerent Boomers

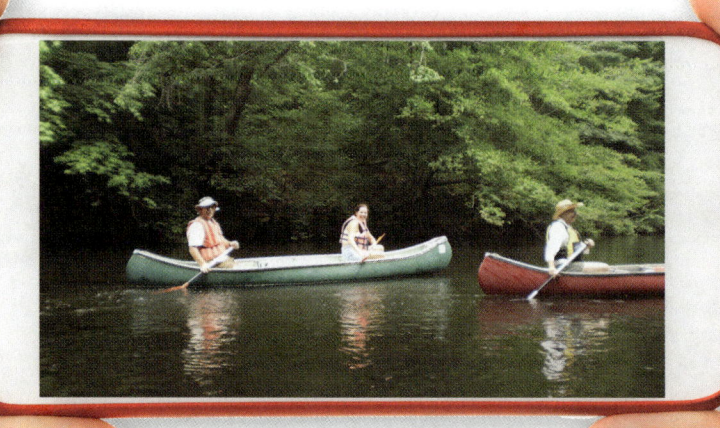

Simple times are the best times.

It boggles the mind when trying to imagine how far technology will take us in the next fifteen years, based on how far we've come just since the dawn of the new millennium.

Smart phones, high speed internet, and GPS systems are

old news by now. I get a little uneasy when I realize my phone is smarter than I am, and I really don't like to think about what is around the next bend.

I overheard a news broadcast this week about a headset being developed which will allow us to post pictures on the internet using only our concentration. You think it, then it magically appears. I hate to think that some of the things I THINK could somehow post themselves on the internet. How embarrassing would that be?

Someone else suggested we will soon have computer strips embedded in our wrists which we will simply slide over a scanner to make purchases at the store. Will currency even be necessary any longer? I think not.

It is projected that self-driving cars could become a reality in the next five years, which tickles me to death. That is most reassuring since I've been dreading that inevitable day my children try to take my keys away. Can flying cars and synthetic brains be far behind? But do you really want someone flying around in your air space who can barely drive down on the ground?

Will space tourism replace Disney World as the hottest destination for vacationers? The medical front is primed for some unbelievable advances. Apparently a device is being developed which will allow your doctor to shake your hand and instantly monitor all your vital signs and take a CT scan. By 2040, it is believed we will be able to download the entire contents of our brains. I'd pass on that because I'm not sure there's very much up there worth downloading.

Personally, I'd rather see technology produce more practical applications. How about a coffee maker that doesn't dribble, or a self-cleaning car that changes its own oil? Maybe a joy stick zapper so we can virtually deliver a big thump on the head to any politician bloviating on television? That would be fun.

> I overheard a news broadcast this week about a headset being developed which will allow us to post pictures on the internet using only our concentration. You think it, then it magically appears. I hate to think that some of the things I THINK could somehow post themselves on the internet. How embarrassing would that be?

How about an automatic rain-maker that can start and stop with a remote control? Why can't they come up with a laser gun which can break up a hurricane or tornado before it destroys an entire city? Now, that's what I'd like to see.

For sure we need a dome to put over the planet to replace the ozone layer. Given the choice, I still prefer the 50s and 60s before cell phones and computers began to monopolize our lives and cut into quality time with our family and friends.

You watch: there will be a drive to cart baby boomers off to "granny pods" to live out their golden years. Well, *au contraire* for my little band of Belligerent Boomers—we have our own plan. We are going to buy a big antebellum home where we will each have a room. There will be a staff to serve our every need including a butler, a driver, a chef, a personal trainer … and a bartender to serve up cocktails on the veranda whenever the clock strikes five somewhere in the world.

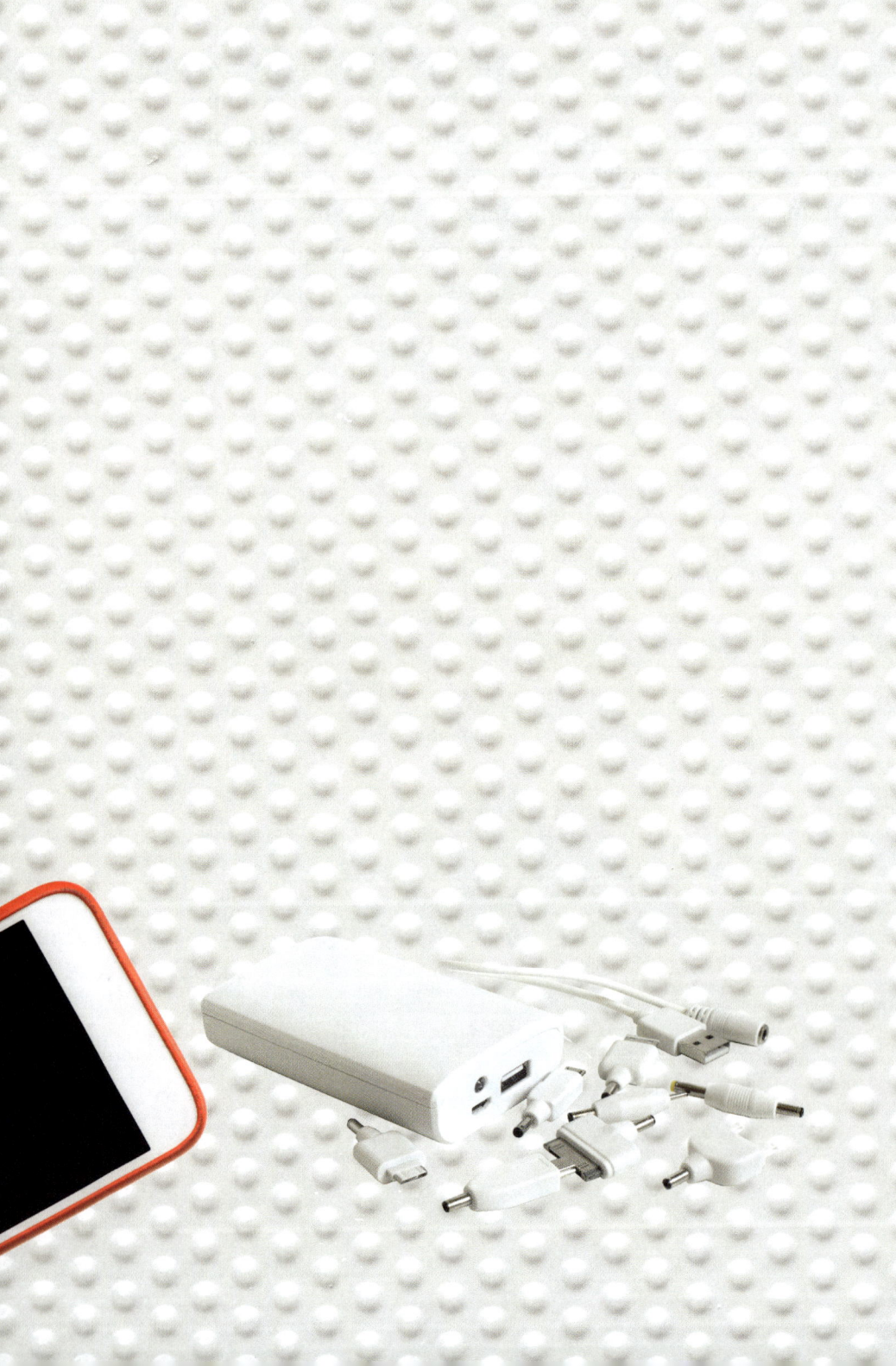

The Awesome

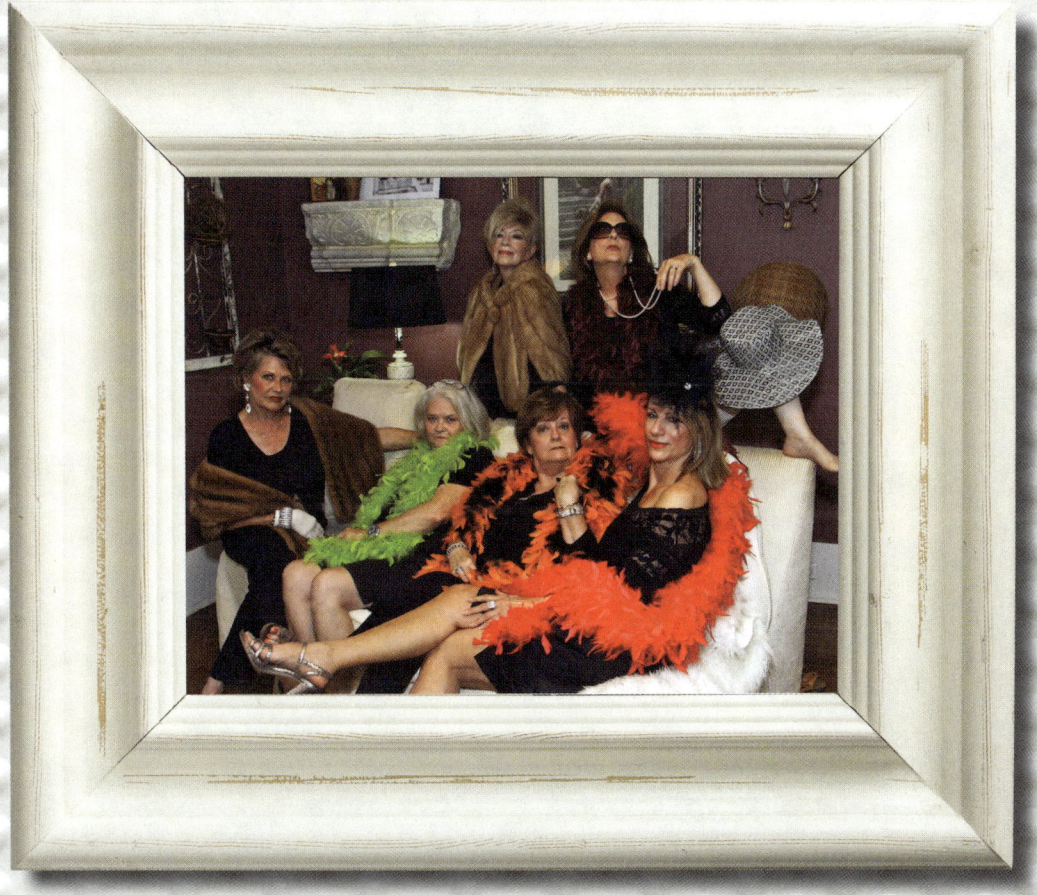

If we think we look good, who cares what anybody else thinks?

Power of Prayer

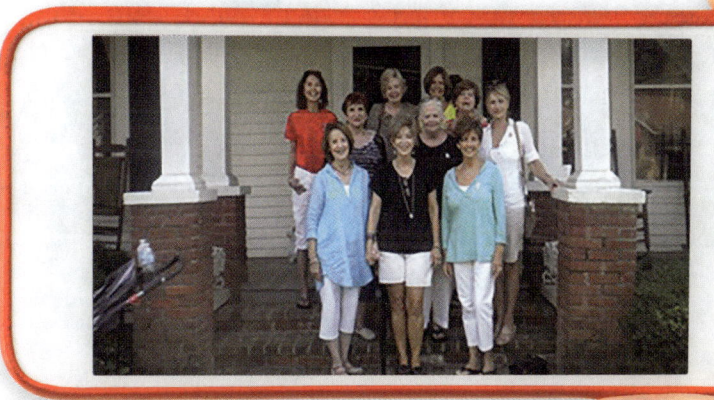

Olivia, front left, has become our very own guardian angel.

I'm wondering if this was my day for Olivia to pray for me. Let me explain.

Each year, Olivia, my lifelong friend who has remained close for sixty-plus years, places all her birthday and Christmas cards in a big bowl. She selects one each day and spends the next twenty-four hours praying for the sender. You can bet she is at the top of the greeting card list for the rest of our tribe, who had the good fortune of graduating from West Point High School together in the 60s.

Good things always happen on the day Olivia prays for us. Some think it is all in our minds, but I don't think so. I think something magical is at work.

Norma, another of our gang, told me she had her day earlier in the week and that her grandson's baseball team, "The Mississippi Longhorns," won the state championship. Norma and I are convinced Olivia had something to do with this.

> ● ● ●
>
> Good things always happen on the day Olivia prays for us. Some think it is all in our minds, but I don't think so. I think something magical is at work.

Anyhow, I arrived home late last night, tired and cranky after being on the road for a total of twenty hours in the last two days attending funerals and new home christenings. Imagine my dismay in discovering that my air conditioner had bitten the dust … again. The interior thermometer read 91 degrees, and I took a bath without even running the hot water.

It was too late to call for help, so I spent one lousy night in late June in a sweaty coma, tossing and turning in a bed that felt like hot ashes. The ceiling fan did little more than circulate the dust particles. Even Lucky Dawg and Rebel were sweating and peered at me with big, sad, moonlike eyes that begged me to do something.

This morning I called my trusty AC repairman. We have become fast friends and sometimes I even fix lunch for him when he's making his calls to tweak my lemon of an air conditioning unit. He's a magician. He always gets me up and running in a matter of minutes at a minimum cost. This time he wouldn't even let me pay him for his time. I think I've become the pity person on his client list.

Now I'm cool as a cucumber, and I got a note from *Publishers Clearinghouse* informing me that I was in the running to win millions. I had a great hair day and found a shirt on sale for two dollars. I called Olivia, and sure enough, this was my day for her to intervene with prayer *just for me*. I knew it! I couldn't think of a single thing that had gone wrong.

I'm off to the store to buy a new supply of greeting cards for every occasion, and many of them are earmarked for the Portera residence in Tuscaloosa, Alabama. I think I may start up this tradition myself. I'd love to get something in my mailbox besides bills and circulars.

Good memory list grows longer everyday

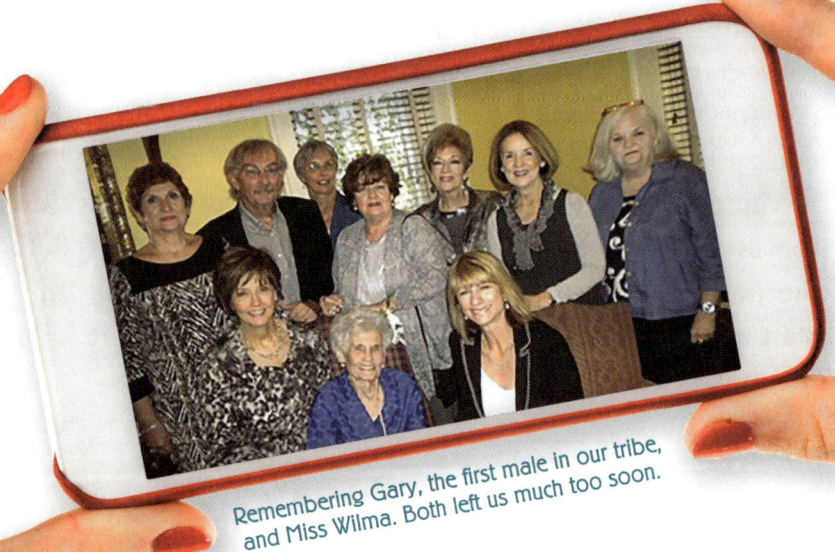

Remembering Gary, the first male in our tribe, and Miss Wilma. Both left us much too soon.

As the years fly by, remembering where I put my car keys has become a challenge, but the memories of growing up in Small Town, Mississippi, are as crisp and clear as a summer morning. I like to think of aging as "selective memory making"—we keep the good and mentally burn the bad.

Today, as temperatures hover around ninety, my thoughts take me back to my childhood when television was not a 24/7 presence and the term *personal computer* was still two decades away. Telephones were all land lines—what else could they possibly be? Some of my friends were lucky enough to have what we called party lines, where several families shared a line and you could eavesdrop on your neighbor's conversations. That was loads of fun.

You've probably figured out by now that I've been infected with a new disease called Acute Nostalgia. As far as I know, there is no treatment or relief from the condition … except to spend as much time as possible with others afflicted by the syndrome. That pretty much includes anyone who grew up in the 50s and 60s and remembers clothes blowing in the wind on the clothesline out back and playing hide-and-go-seek at dusk. You could be decapitated by those same clotheslines as you darted across the neighbor's backyard to get back to home base.

In those days everybody loved Lucy and Father knew best. We would make ourselves a Coke float, sit on the davenport, and hum along with the dreamy guys, singing *Do Wah Diddy Diddy*. Good art in those days was framed prints of dogs playing poker.

I loved watching Dinah Shore sing "See the USA in your Chevrolet" when the average cost of the family car was a mere $2,749, and—brace yourself—gasoline was only 24 cents a gallon! A guy once told me that a car with fins guaranteed him a date with the cutest girl in the class.

But there was much more to the 50s than sock hops and milkshakes delivered to your car window by a girl wearing skates. For one thing, there was no swearing on TV. In fact, there was no swearing in life. I was once grounded for a week for saying DANG IT, and that's no lie. (I only say *no lie* because it has come to my attention that some people think I make this stuff up.) I was grounded for two weeks—TWO WEEKS!—for sneaking into a limited showing of *Splendor in the Grass*. Oh, the shame!

"One of our favorite activities in the 50s was holding 'Communion' in the ditch that ran underneath the street where I grew up. We would sneak grape juice and crackers to crush and ceremoniously munch on while tossing back a jigger of juice. We also made "snuff" on a regular basis by mixing cocoa and sugar and stuffing it in our top lips, letting the juice run down our cheeks. I still get the urge to do that today."

—Emily B. Jones

Those were the days when the whole family sat down for dinner every night at a table and occupied the very same pew in church each Sunday. Heaven help the stranger who wandered in and dared sit in your place. Incidentally, it was true what the rest of the world thought about us hicks in the south—we didn't wear shoes from May to September except for Sundays, and there was no pain like being caught in a patch of stickers on a hot summer afternoon. You could miss supper waiting for someone to come rescue you. And we had supper every evening. Dinner was always at twelve noon.

My nose remained sunburned from May to September, and I fully expect to come down with skin cancer any day now. We lounged around in the sun wearing a homemade suntan lotion concocted from baby oil and iodine. Why in the world would you want something called sunscreen? That was counterintuitive to our 50s way of thinking. The whole point was to sport a nice healthy glow (while being oblivious to the dangers). Thankfully we can now get that glow out of a bottle—and on a cloudy day.

We had just been introduced to the Frisbee and the hula hoop, and to coin a phrase, it was a very good year for small town girls and soft summer nights. We'd hide from the lights on the village green when I was seventeen. (Wait, maybe I didn't coin that phrase after all.)

My mother planted pine trees in the front yard, which were in perfect alignment for our bases during an afternoon game of softball. I still remember her yelling at us to stop pulling needles off those precious pines. After she died, Daddy had to have those trees cut because he was afraid a high wind would blow them onto the house.

My best friends and closest neighbors, Phil, Martha, Lota, Margaret, Heard, and Larry would have "fop fights" every Saturday morning. In case you haven't had the pleasure, a fop fight is when you take all the leftover copies of the *Daily Times Leader* from Phil's paper route, wet them down, and pummel each other until you're black and blue. Boy, was that fun or what? Martha is gone now, and the rest of us have joined the ranks of retiree. How did it happen so fast?

But the memories come flooding back when I hear the buzzing of a bee, which is a rarity these days. Where have all the bees gone? And the frogs. They were everywhere in the 50s and the boys used to taunt us with them. The worst feeling in the world was when Phil would put one down my tank top. (Incidentally, the wearing of a tank top on this fifty-something body will occur about the time evolution eliminates the human little toe.)

So what do you remember about your childhood? What sparks your return to the child who still lurks inside? I wonder if your memories are similar to mine and half as wonderful. I feel like the luckiest woman in the world to have been allowed to grow up in Small Town USA, where all the women are strong, all the men are good-looking, and all the children were above average. (Ah, a little plagiarism never hurts a writer's style, especially if her credibility is questionable anyway.)

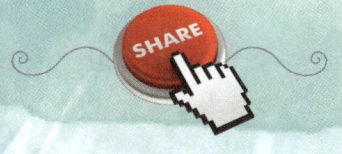

Rock On, Boomers

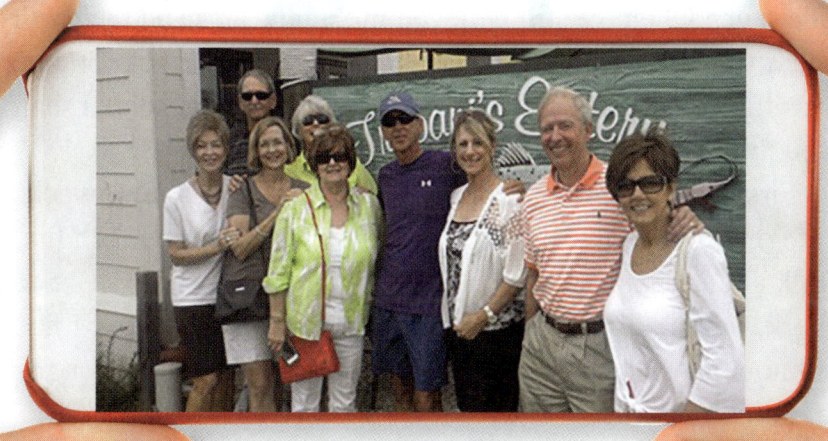

Several times a year we cruise the Coast
with our tribe. The coastal residents
probably dread it.

Being a card carrying member of the first wave of baby boomers to appear on the planet, I feel fortunate to still be breathing.

Suddenly, without warning, people have begun referring to the entire Boomer Nation as (gulp) senior citizens.

Whoa! Not so fast, you folks who still have pigment in your

hair. I prefer the term "chronologically gifted." Didn't you get the memo that the age bracket for seniors has officially been adjusted upward, so 60 is the new 40? (I wish someone would tell my sciatic nerve.)

But I must say that aging has come with some delightful perks, especially the rediscovery of good, old-fashioned fun. Maybe there is justice in the world after all.

I'm not talking about the grown-up kind of fun we had in our 30s and 40s which involved bringing home a fat paycheck or airline tickets to some foreign land. It's the kind we had at age seven when we still believed in Santa Claus and the tooth fairy. Giving the dog a bath or painting your bicycle orange was fun back then. And trust me, it will be again, sooner than you think.

First you've got to reorder your priorities. A few weeks into retirement I discovered I wasn't having all that much fun. Talk about depressing. All I had done for 40 years was go to work, raise children, and do some short-order cooking. I had no hobbies and no simple pleasures ... well, except for my morning coffee.

I had a few friends—the same ones I had worked with—and they were now too busy to go drag-racing with me. With an abundance of free time and a calendar that wasn't full of to-dos (like saving the world), I actually stumbled across the ability to have fun again.

But first I had to be willing to toss caution to the wind and break the rules. Go ahead and block out your mother's voice and take candy from strangers, and by all means wear white shoes after Labor Day. Heck, I wore white shoes today—with pink socks. (The younger generation expects us to be tacky, and I can do tacky.)

You can paint your guest room fuchsia, then take the left-over paint outside and paint big floppy flowers on your fence. You can purchase a tiara at the toy store and wear it to the supermarket. I never got to be a beauty queen, but I can now wear my new tiara to the Piggly Wiggly and attract all kinds of strange people to add to my "new friends" list.

You can still be the life of the party even if the party ends by 8 p.m.

If you find yourself rusty in the fun category, try this: set a timer, and for ten minutes write down all the things you'd like to do, as fast as you can, and without editing. Don't think, just write. Don't judge and don't give yourself time to wonder if it will get you incarcerated or make you a laughing stock.

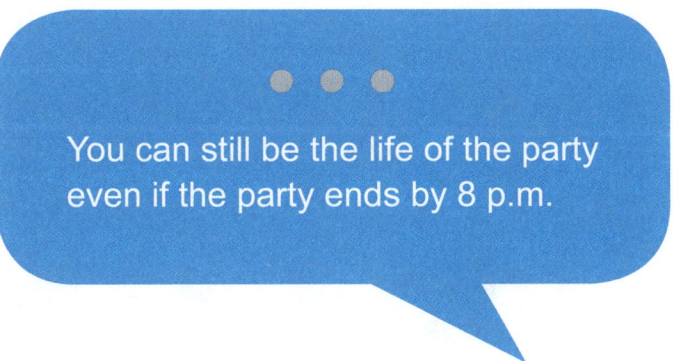

You can still be the life of the party even if the party ends by 8 p.m.

Let the thoughts fly onto the page as fast as your brain can spit them out. My list included pouring a whole bottle of bubble bath into the tub, and making a batch of fudge to share with NO ONE. Eat the fudge in the tub so you don't get all sticky. Think of everything you've ever wanted to do but were repressed by decorum.

When your ten minutes of listing are up, pick two items and do them. You will acquire a daring new attitude and your list will keep growing. Suddenly, every day becomes a great adventure and you'll make friends with other emancipated people.

Never forget that people, like fine wine, become more valuable with age. I'm just hoping I'm not a bottle of Ripple.

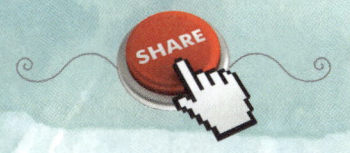

Pain killer that doesn't require a prescription

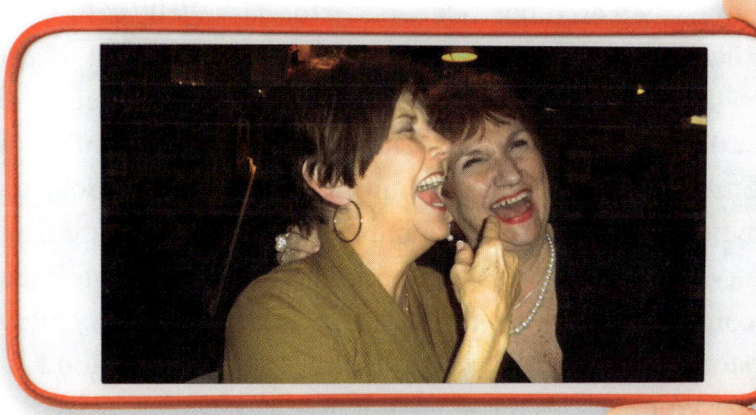

If laughter is a drug, Beth is our dealer.

I have this cousin. Bill Poe is his name. Well, he's not really my cousin, but we pretend we are—it's a long story which I won't go into here because I can't wait to share a brilliant prescription he gave me this week. It's to be used ostensibly in annoying moments, but I'm finding it has multiple applications.

The secret he revealed is a surefire way to defuse those tense, anxious moments which threaten to bring us down. It has worked for me this week in the following situations: when I discovered my hot water heater is leaking and the floor seems a little squishy; when I came home from my temporary job at the local newspaper dog-tired, then discovered we had a hole in the front page the size of Arizona to be filled with news that hadn't happened yet; that nagging voice in my head (that sounds like Ruth Daniel, my CPA) reminding me time is running out to get my taxes together.

I could go on and on, but we all have those little irritants that muddy up an otherwise wonderful day. Well, hold on to your hats, folks. Those days will not be muddied again if you follow a few simple instructions which Bill has perfected.

It all started this week when I was sitting in my office at the *Starkville Daily News* ranting to a co-worker about the annoying practice of using abbreviations for everything from country clubs to government programs. I was asked to meet someone at OWGC in West Point. How could I possibly know that stood for Old Waverly Golf Club? I thought it stood for the Old Women's Gynocology Clinic.

Just when I had worked myself into the stroke zone, Cousin Bill waltzed in and sat down to observe my tirade. He didn't say a word, just looked at me weirdly for a moment then broke out into an evil laughter that sounded like "muahahahahaha." I stared at him in confusion as the laughter grew more intense.

Wait … was a smile forcing its way through my pursed lips? Was there a small rumble of laughter building in my chest and bubbling upward? Within seconds, we were laughing so hard the rest of the staff was peering around the doorway to see if it was time to call for help. The harder and louder Bill laughed, the more determined I was to keep pace. The magic of the moment was that what began as completely forced laughter had mysteriously evolved into the real thing.

> • • •
>
> "Laughter and tears are both responses to frustration and exhaustion. I myself prefer to laugh, since there is less cleaning to do afterwards."
>
> —Kurt Vonnegut

After about five minutes of this, exhausted and completely laughed out, we paused to try to figure out what just happened. "Feel better?" he asked. "Oh yeah," I responded, trying to suppress the remains of one last giggle.

Then he told me a story. Several years ago his family took a cruise. On the ship was an entertainer named David Naster, author of a book entitled, *You Just Have to LAUGH Through Hard Times*.

"The first thing he did was to instruct the audience to turn to your right, look the person in the face, and start laughing," Bill said. "Awkward at first, but moments later the house was roaring in laughter."

"Now," Naster said next to the group, "don't you feel more

relaxed?"

After the cruise, Bill said he often calls family members to have a good laugh whether or not anything is particularly funny.

I can't wait to try this out at the next meeting I'm attending. Laughter is one of the most contagious activities I can think of, and I challenge you to become a carrier.

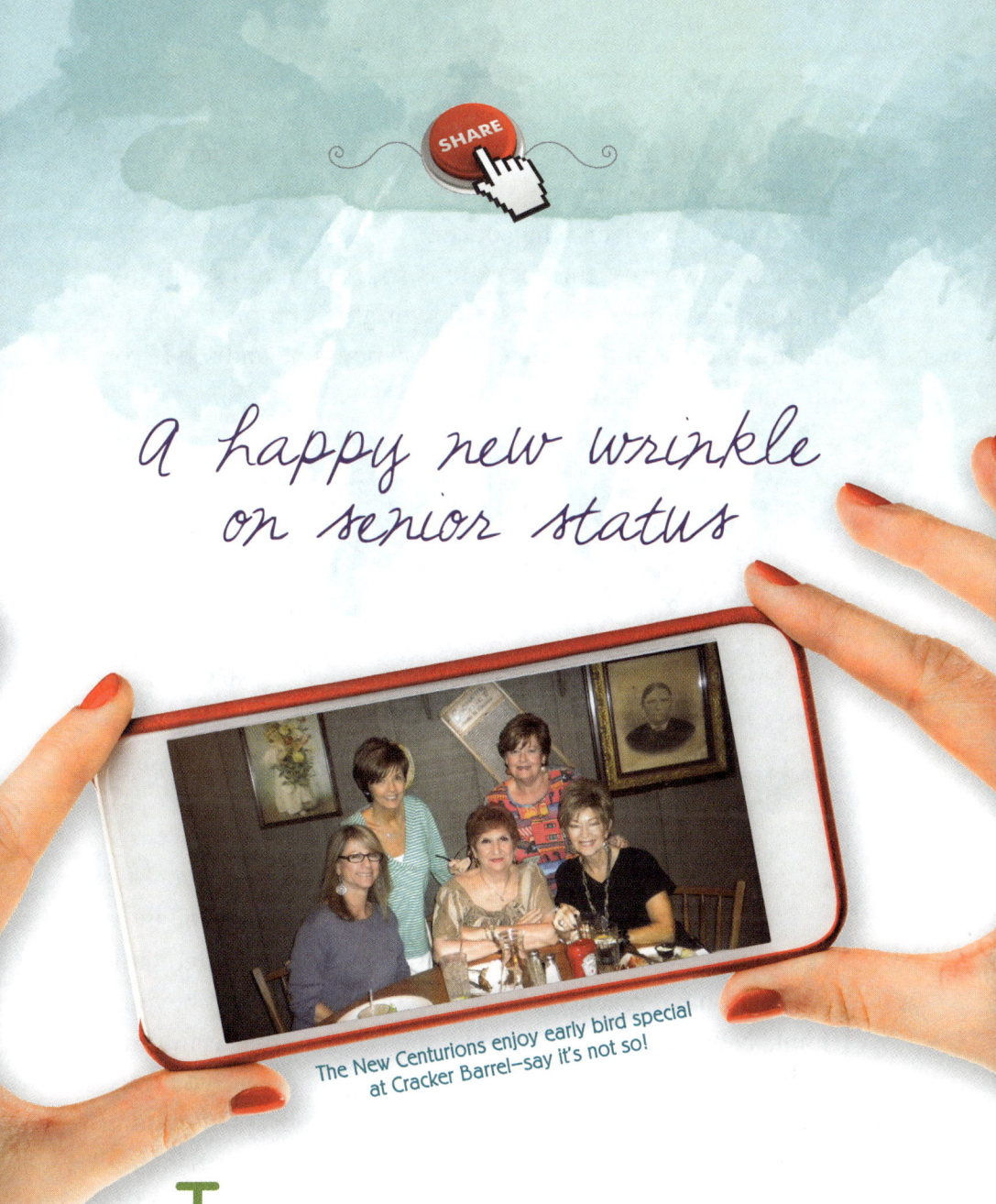

a happy new wrinkle on senior status

The New Centurions enjoy early bird special at Cracker Barrel—say it's not so!

Is your glass half empty or half full? Sometimes the glass is just too blamed big. Or in my case it has a slow leak.

Thinking about that leak, I am organizing a protest for the flagrant insults I see spreading with regard to senior citizen status. First of all, I don't like being called a senior. I was a senior a half century ago at West Point High School and there's no comparison whatsoever.

Hands down, my current state is so much more soul satisfying, and at times it can be downright hilarious. You try dancing in front of the mirror to some pop tune and see if you don't think it's hilarious.

> • • •
>
> Tell your well-meaning younger friends that it is like being kissed and slapped at the same time when they tell you that you look great for your age.

I've been trying to come up with a new term to pigeonhole those who have reached the half century mark and beyond. I think New Centurions sounds courageous, masterful, and highly-evolved. To be over 50 in this day and age, you must be all those things or get lost in this youth-obsessed culture. The New Centurions conjures up visions of a silver-haired siren karate-chopping, then collaring the punk who tried to steal her purse. He won't mess with her again.

Furthermore, I choose to think of my gang as "seasoned adults in their prime"—magnificent even, rather than dim-witted dinosaurs who can't find their cars in the parking lot.

Well, true, I can rarely find my car on the first try, but people half my age have that problem because all vehicles look alike these days (in this white SUV-obsessed culture. I'm shopping for an orange Ferrari to solve that problem and I'm enjoying the test drives immensely).

It may be hard for some to imagine, but every older adult was at one time young and full of energy, passion, ambition, and dreams. We still have goals way beyond completing a small craft project, walking to the mailbox, or finishing our prune juice. I'm tried of late-night comedians joking about us and our memory loss—did you ever consider that we forget some things because we want to? And besides, our brains are so stuffed with facts (both significant and insignificant) that we're obligated to let something go every now and then or our heads would explode.

And enough with the "elder speak"—shouting at us like we can't hear, using a singsong voice, and using the pronoun *we* instead of you. "Are we ready for our applesauce now, dearie?" said one well-meaning caregiver when I was visiting an assisted living facility recently. "We're more ready for a double martini," I replied, and was ignored.

Enough already with this pervading and condescending attitude toward the New Centurions. Every other segment of society is looking for respect, so why not extend it to the brave folks advancing on the enemy (old age) and finding ways to successfully hold it at bay?

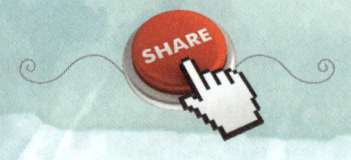

The joy of preparing Granny's recipes

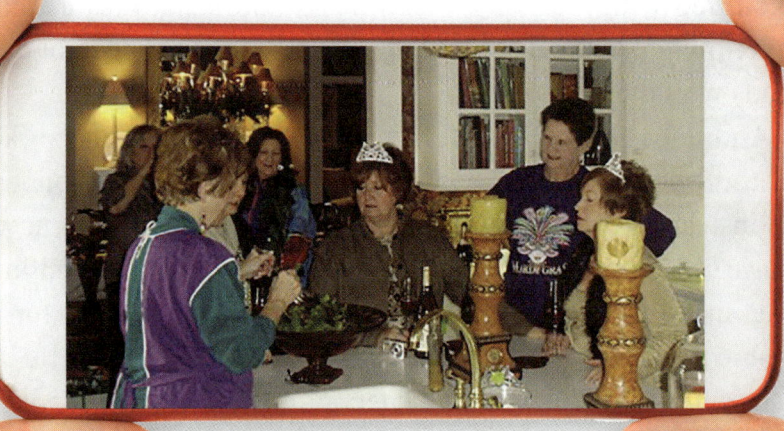

My gang always ends up in the kitchen cooking and eating.

C hildhood memories often lure me into a disappearing world of culinary and sensory delights. Those were the days of anticipation which made you drool when you heard the rotary mixer hit the side of the glass bowl, or the popping of grease from the frying pan (which heralded a batch of fried chicken).

Or, oh my, the smell of a pie fresh-baked from the oven with a homemade crust. I haven't had one of those since the Eisenhower administration.

These days I just buy a candle called Apple Pie Spice and plop a bucket of KFC on the table beside bottles of designer water. Those olfactory culinary pleasantries of yesteryear are likely to cause a panic attack among the self-declared food police who have taken all the fun out of eating. Frying anything is considered gauche; lard has become the devil incarnate; the mixer is dying of boredom because everyone is avoiding the sugary desserts which require one.

Entertaining has become a nightmare, because in my circle of friends and family everyone is either vegan, gluten-free, lactose intolerant, suffering from acid reflux, or worried about animal rights. Counting carbs is more fashionable than calories and suddenly the lowly potato is in danger of extinction. I'm almost glad Granny never had to see such a travesty.

Cooking has become a challenge of monumental proportions, especially during the holidays when you strive to accommodate every taste and ban all things judged unhealthy by someone in Washington. Ordering a salad when you really want a burger has become a badge of honor, and depriving ourselves is a national pastime. So why as a nation have we become fatter? Could it be we're sharing our beds with a package of Oreos after everyone goes home?

I can see my grandmother's table groaning under platters of mashed potatoes swimming in gravy, corn on the cob picked at its peak and flash frozen last summer, peas cooked in bacon drippings, and the best cornbread dressing this side of the Mississippi. She would have cringed at my table laden with some unidentifiable substance called tofu, a newfangled grain called quinoa (pronounced Keen-wa), and Stove Top stuffing mix. Oh, the horror!

> • • •
>
> "Food is therapy for most of us during these difficult times. And when I think 'comfort food' I really mean rich gooey dishes that instantly release dopamine and serotonin into the brain, and suddenly you forget about the 3,000 calories you just consumed."
>
> —Emily B. Jones

The food prepared by my grandmother was simple fare, and to date has never been replicated outside her blue and white-checkered kitchen. Her menu always included squash and onions fried in bacon drippings, long-simmered collards mingled with white chunks of turnips (and dressed in hot-pepper vinegar), and butterbeans cooked down to creamy heaps. These dishes were eaten before the main event, which was pecan pie (if the trees produced that year; egg custard if they didn't). Prepared pie shells wouldn't come along until the middle of the twentieth century.

My grandmother's spice cabinet contained salt, pepper, cinnamon, and vanilla. That was it. I doubt she ever heard of cumin or dried basil. And Rosemary was the name of her second cousin.

While trying to live healthier lives and trim the extra pounds, food became the enemy somewhere around 1980 when processed food emerged as a cheaper alternative to fresh fruits and vegetables.

We live in an age when professional cooks are household names, and some of them are as famous as athletes or movie stars. We spend more time watching food being cooked on television than we spend actually cooking it. We are so incredibly blessed as a nation, but I can't help but feel we have sacrificed the tastiest of creature comforts to conform to the latest designer fare.

Right now I'm cooking up chicken and dumplings like my grandmother used to make, and it looks like the kitchen got hit with the first snow of the season. Now I remember why I don't cook from scratch—cleaning up is too taxing. But once in a blue moon I will continue to try … just so I don't forget how to do it.

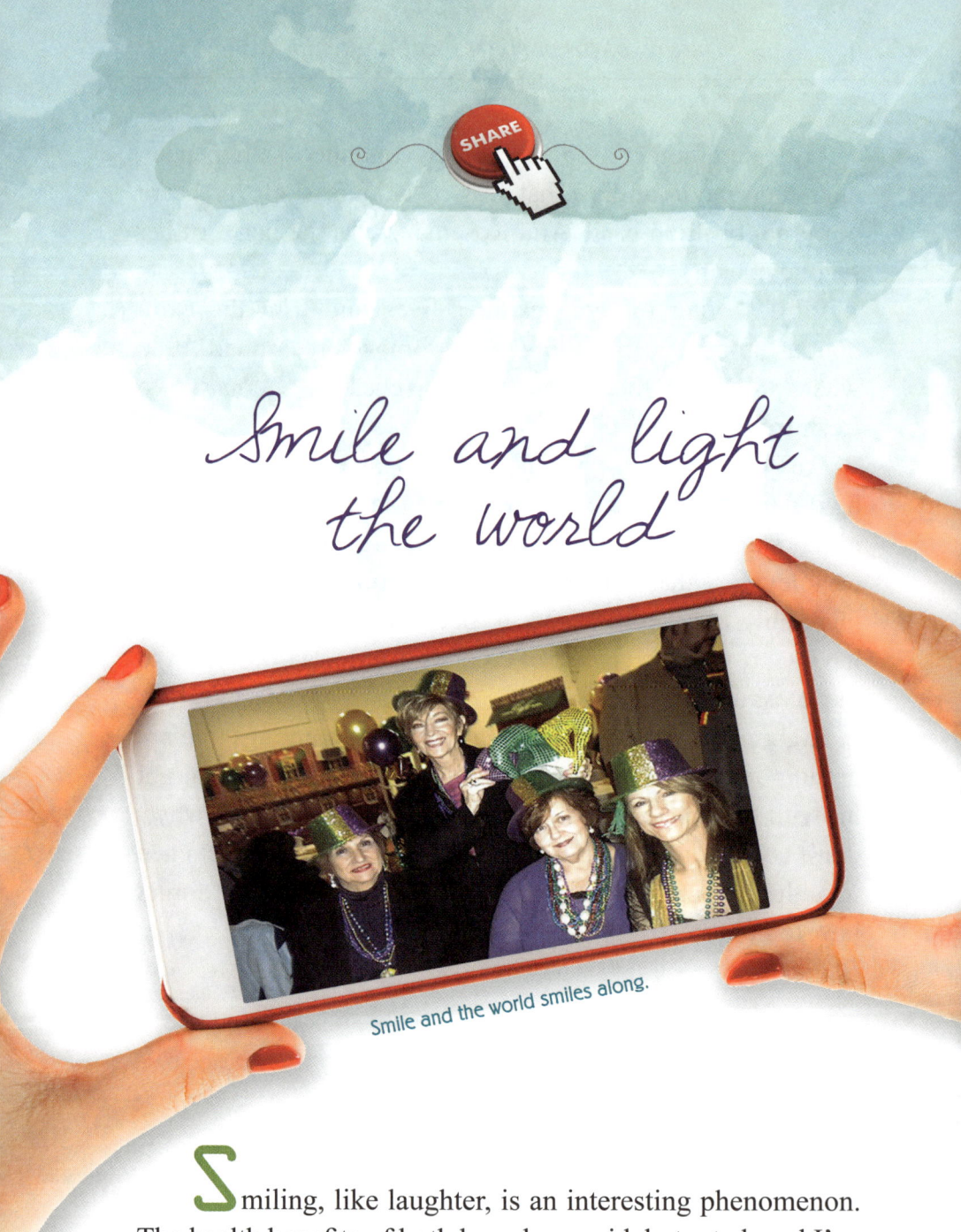

Smile and light the world

Smile and the world smiles along.

Smiling, like laughter, is an interesting phenomenon. The health benefits of both have been widely touted, and I've written previously about the pain-relieving aspects of laughter, but I never thought much about smiling. It seems almost involuntary and is one activity which bridges all cultural and age barriers.

Studies suggest that smiling, forced or not, can have a positive effect on our mood, decrease stress levels, and make everyone around you feel better. What happy news!

Oh, and studies show that people who smile a lot are considered more attractive than their straight-faced companions. (By now you must be grinning ear to ear—I know I am.)

While waiting in a doctor's office this week for well over an hour, I began to think I'd never smile again; patience is not one of my virtues. To distract myself I picked up a magazine from a stack of male-oriented reading materials. I selected a periodical on psychology (because it was either that or *Popular Mechanics*) and opened it right up to a piece on the value of a smile. I smiled in spite of my agitation.

Get this: The article said we need to increase our daily diet of genuine smiles not only to get along with our peers, but for psychological and physical health as well. It stated that we humans need three positive emotions to lift us up for every one negative emotion that wears us down. So, I calculated that we need three or more smiles for each grimace.

By then, I was griming like a loon to see if it would serve as a balm to my thinning patience. Everyone around me peered over their glasses suspiciously—as if I were about to pull a gun from my pantyhose and go on a shooting spree. But soon, they began smiling back. The atmosphere in the whole room changed in an instant and we began small talk … which quickly grew into large talk! We were sick people wallowing in self-pity one minute, and a bunch of co-conspirators laughing about our infirmities the next.

We've been baring our teeth—I suppose—since the

beginning of time. I read somewhere that cavemen smiled big ole toothy grins for potential mates to prove they had good teeth. I don't know about that, but I bet he got his girl and they smiled happily ever after.

In my experience, a smile is typically a response to someone else's smile, since a well-placed smile is extremely contagious and can often lead to a lovely conversation. And if we're lucky, a laugh or two.

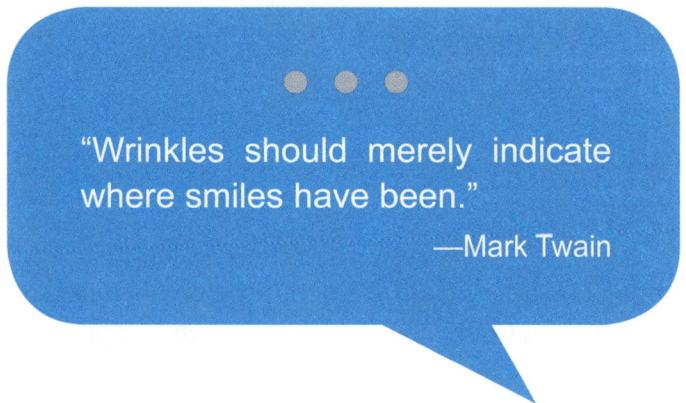

"Wrinkles should merely indicate where smiles have been."
—Mark Twain

But there is a difference in a faked smile and the genuine grin which requires parts of the whole face to be convincing. There is a woman on one of the morning network news shows who grins a lot—but I suspect she is unhappy because her eyes remain uninvolved. I call her Dead Eyes, but to be fair she has probably had Botox (which renders parts of the face impervious to emotion). That's why I will never go that route, and will instead spend thousands on every miracle cream pitched on the internet and the Home Shopping Network.

Many years ago, I did radio commercials for an ad agency. One day when I was not delivering my lines very convincingly, the technician suggested that I smile while reading from the script. That simple act totally changed the tone of the lines, which transformed the whole feeling of the commercial from drab to colorful!

One thing I know for sure: the world looks brighter from behind a smile, and a brilliant smile can defuse the tensest of situations. And remember this: If you would like to spoil the day for a grouch, give him a big ole smile.

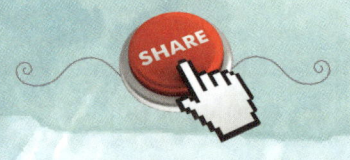

Hooray, sweat pants became a fashion statement

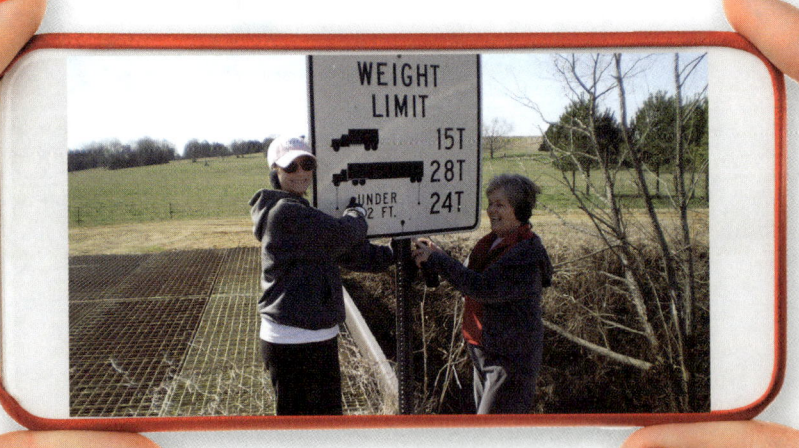

Sweats—wear them proudly—you can
always pretend you are training for
the marathon.

Today I went to Walmart to pick up a new lipstick and left
with some key pieces for my senior citizen wardrobe. On a
whim I wandered into the clothing section to see if the sweat
pants and matching shirts might be on sale. Since we're near

the end of the harshest winter in my memory, my uniform (a.k.a. my sweats wardrobe) is permanently tattooed with chili stains and puppy throw-up. (Feeding the leftover chili to pets is never a good idea.)

Indeed, the sweats were on sale. (I've been watching a lot of British television on Netflix and have adopted a slight British accent, therefore finding myself saying things like "indeed" when agreeing with something and, "May I have a word?" (pronounced '*wod*') when I want someone's attention). But that's a story for another day. Today I'm on a soapbox for that fleecy, stretchy, comfort wear which is so maligned by the fashionistas.

Sweatpants get a bad rap for being frumpy and best reserved for the comfort of your own home or the gym. Designer Karl Lagerfeld has been quoted as saying, "Sweatpants are a sign of defeat. You lose control of your life so you buy some sweatpants." Indeed, Mr. Lagerfeld. With all due respect, could it be your need to put down the lowly sweats to sell your designer jeans and jackets which are so expensive they require mortgage financing?

I concede that you probably don't want to wear sweatpants to a job interview or your best friend's wedding, but I think there are plenty of occasions outside the home or gym when they are perfectly acceptable.

I'm tired of sweatpants and shirts being the pit bull of the fashion world, both feared and misunderstood. I think people associate them with laziness and sloth, but that's just wrong. I, for one, work best when I am comfortable, and I am most comfortable in my sweats. I secretly pine for my fleecy, go-to wardrobe while stuffing myself into pencil skirts or skin-tight jeans which can only be zipped while reclining.

Most people just want to be comfortable in forgiving clothing which can enable them to eat three pieces of lemon icebox pie without having their circulation cut off. There's a reassuring quality to a well-worn pair of sweats. You can sleep in them on a cold winter night and roll out the next morning and dash to the Piggly Wiggly for donuts if you're being bad, or broccoli if you're being good.

> • • •
>
> My new favorite author had this explanation for going out in public without bothering with her appearance: "If I did not wear a stained sweatshirt, orthopaedic shoes, and have frantically disheveled hair, I would be so beautiful men would go mad—married men would run amok."
>
> —Brenda Ueland

Sweats offer the non-judgmental comfort of flannel pajamas while creating the illusion that aerobic activity is on the horizon. While in the Piggly Wiggly, I tell everyone I just dashed in for some bottled water to take to my workout at the gym. Since I'm already there, I pick up the things I really need and no one's the wiser.

Another good thing about sweatpants is that they're cheap. Toward the end of the season you can pick up three pairs for $20. Or, if designer clothing is your thing, the trendy Juicy Couture brand can set you back as much as $250 for a set of velour-hooded sweats. I'm sticking with my Hanes from Walmart, even though they tend to "pill-up" on you after several hundred washings. The pants also grow shorter with each washing until you have some baggy shorts just in time for spring. What could be more practical?

Did you know that sweats have been around since the 1920s, when they were introduced in France? Yup, sweats are French! In my opinion they rank right up there with French fries, penicillin, and the polio vaccine as society's most important developments.

Sweats could even be critical to your health. The human body has 2-4 million sweat glands, which enable us to cool down and maintain proper body temperature. Shouldn't sweats be encouraged rather than ostracized?

Since the introduction of Casual Fridays, sweat suits have become a tad more socially acceptable, and I'm hoping they will eventually morph into a fashion statement for Mousy Mondays, Sloppy Saturdays, and Slumming Sundays. After all, life is too short to "sweat" the small stuff, like what we are wearing—especially if it itches, pinches, squeezes, or pulls. I've never met a pair of sweats I didn't love.

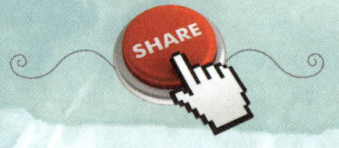

Cry me a river, please!

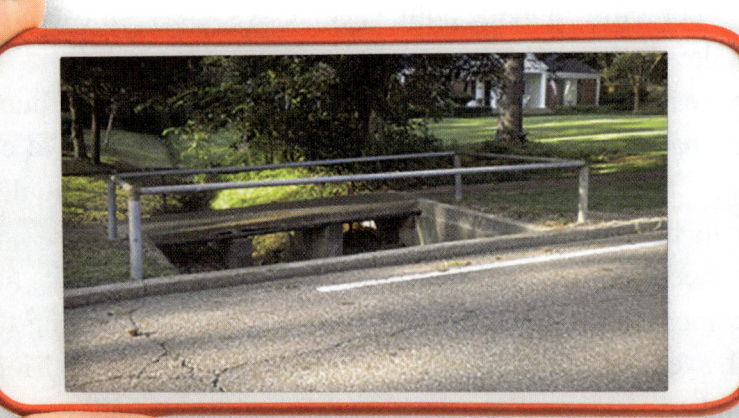

Regardless of where we got our degrees, our real education was acquired playing in a drainage ditch which ran beside my house in West Point, Mississippi.

Have you ever been so deliriously happy that for some inexplicable reason, tears welled up in your eyes and meandered down your cheeks along with your eye makeup? You looked like something from *Halloween II* while everyone looked at you with pity—as if you'd lost your dog or something equally tragic?

Well, I've been crying for the last three days. My eyes are swollen and the emotions I'm wearing on my sleeve are maroon, white, red, and blue. I've read about tears of joy, but I've not experienced such ecstasy since the birth of my children.

It all began at Davis Wade Stadium last Saturday afternoon when the Mississippi State Bulldogs gave Auburn a good *whuppin*. Fans, packed into the stadium like sardines, were hugging, high-fiving, and jumping up and down. Me? I was standing there bawling like a baby and I don't even understand the finer points of the game. I just like getting dressed up in school colors and watching people in the stadium. Not this time, sports fans. I watched every play and even spotted an Auburn player clip one of our guys. (A week ago I thought a clip was a hair utensil.)

Later that evening, we watched the Rebels pummel Texas A&M almost as soundly as the Dawgs did the week before. I sat there with tears bubbling out my nose. It was a beautiful thing to behold, watching the State and Ole Miss players operate as a unit, all for one and one for all—making Mississippians around the world drop what they were doing and feel a part of this supreme coup.

On Sunday morning I watched an ESPN special on Dak Prescott and my heart almost exploded. Entitled *Faith, Family and Football*, he explained his philosophy of life with humility and clarity befitting a true hero. If he doesn't win the Heisman, something is terribly wrong with the system.

Of course, out-and-out sobbing began on Sunday when the new Coaches poll was released. The Dawgs had arrived at that elusive NUMBER ONE IN THE NATION slot with the Rebels close behind. Who could have imagined such a thing only weeks ago? The implications of all this extends way beyond the gridiron. They won't have Mississippi to kick around any more.

Mississippi has character born of adversity and resolved in the love of our teams which are composed of us all. Pride and joy have brought all the state's diverse groups together with a common voice, and we adore this group of young players who have achieved what no politician or special interest group could ever accomplish.

Mississippi has character born of adversity and resolved in the love of our teams which are composed of us all. Pride and joy have brought all the state's diverse groups together with a common voice, and we adore this group of young players who have achieved what no politician or special interest group could ever accomplish.

Exquisitely beautiful and somewhat surprising to me were the reactions of both Coach Mullen and Coach Freeze. Mullen, a man after my own heart, teared up—while Freeze was so excited he fell down on the sidelines in *America's Funniest Home Videos* fashion.

The Clarion-Ledger delivered the icing on the cake when they named my book *Love, Laughter & Losing My Keys: A Survival Guide for Baby Boomers* to the Top Ten reads in Mississippi (excuse the blatant brag). The book beat out Bill O'Reilly's *Killing Patton*. Never in my wildest dreams could I imagine any of this. I figure people are weary of pestilence and ready for some lighthearted fun.

Isn't it ironic that it took Mississippi State and Ole Miss to show the world how it should be done.

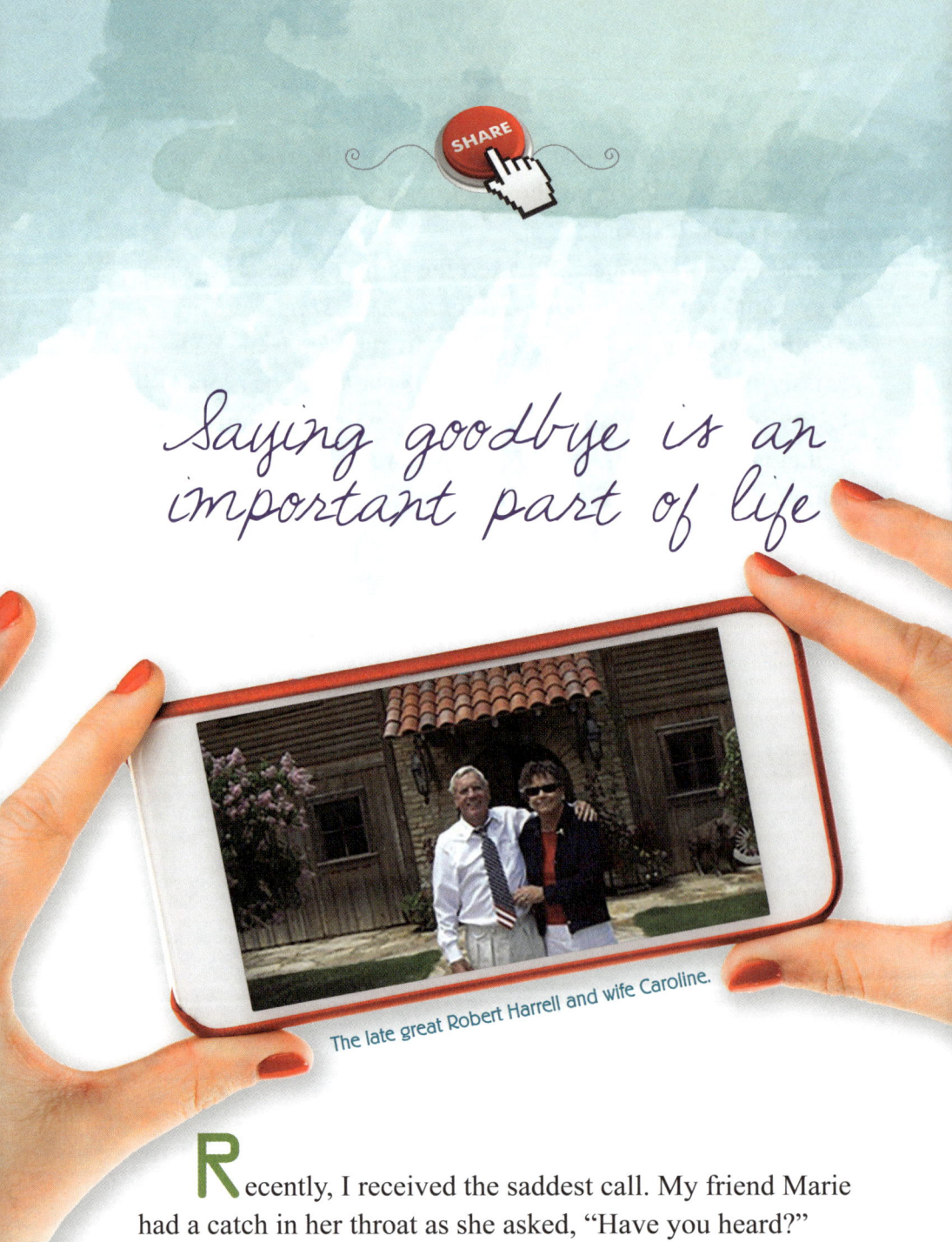

Saying goodbye is an important part of life

The late great Robert Harrell and wife Caroline.

Recently, I received the saddest call. My friend Marie had a catch in her throat as she asked, "Have you heard?"

I'd heard that same catch in her throat two years ago when she called to tell us our friend Gary had died. I knew what was coming was going to be bad, so I braced myself for the saddest news I've heard since I lost my mother back in 1977.

Robert Harrell, an indescribable man and a friend to everyone he ever met, died Monday after a car accident in our hometown of West Point, Mississippi. There was a question as to whether he had suffered some sort of medical episode which caused the wreck. I don't know the details and this is not an obituary, just a few thoughts on a remarkable man who had a positive impact on so many lives. To say he aged well is an understatement.

Many Robert Harrell stories are included in my last book *Love, Laughter & Losing My Keys*. He was an inspiration and a role model on how to live life fully with vitality and unbridled joy. In fact, I never saw him without a huge grin on his face, and he possessed an endearing quality that made everyone he met feel like the most important person on earth.

Robert was brilliant. Seriously, I think of him as West Point's Leonardo da Vinci because he had a curiosity about everything. He had many interests and pursued them tirelessly, never considering that anything was impossible.

He was to be our guide when we hike the Appalachian Trail because he's done it and we couldn't think of anyone more fun to help complete our bucket list. His death reminds me to stop putting off our dreams before it's too late. Hiking the trail no longer holds such promise of a first-rate adventure without Robert along to keep us entertained.

My favorite memory was one sultry July afternoon when Robert drove Daddy and me in his golf cart out into the woods surrounding his house to show off what I've begun thinking of as Robert's World. He kept up a running dialogue of fascinating tidbits of trivia: explaining the length of a furlong and what the abbreviation "cc" means on a prescription bottle. Important stuff like that.

The legendary Robert Harrell was giving us a tour of what amounts to an amusement park. At least it was an amusement to Robert, its owner and developer, who built a small community in the woods surrounding his Old Waverly Road home.

> • • •
>
> Robert was brilliant. Seriously, I think of him as West Point's Leonardo da Vinci because he had a curiosity about everything. He had many interests and pursued them tirelessly, never considering that anything was impossible.

As long as I can remember, I've been the recipient and distributor of Robert Harrell stories, some so far-fetched I couldn't believe they were true. If you had the good fortune to grow up in Clay County, Mississippi, it was practically a requirement to carry in your head a couple of Robert Harrell stories to pull out whenever a conversation hit a lull.

My thoughts and prayers are with his wife of a gazillion years, Caroline, and all their children. I remember when Robert and Caroline were teenagers and I was around ten. My friend Olivia and I would jockey for a seat behind them at church so we could observe and dream of the day we would find our own Robert. Unfortunately it hasn't happened yet for me because there is no other Robert.

I tell you all this to remind myself that losing dear friends and family members is the hardest part of life. That's why we should never miss the opportunity to say "I love you" to those we love while they can still hear us.

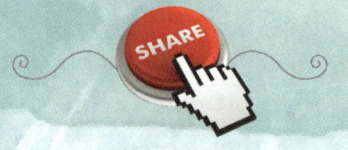

What I love about growing older (seriously)

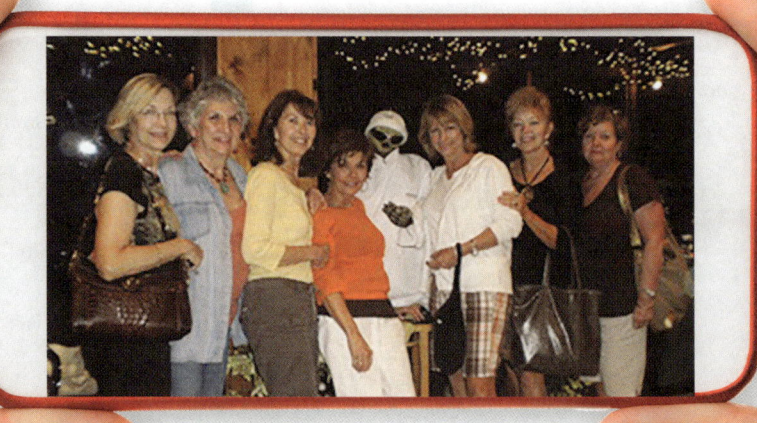

The best part is traveling with friends.
(We have no idea who that weird guy is in
the middle of the photo. We're pretty sure
he's an extraterrestrial.)

L et's face it. From the moment we're born, we're growing older. But don't expect me to commiserate about the negatives of the condition. I choose instead to dwell on the good side of aging, and I find more to appreciate with each passing year.

Okay, so I'm the queen of denial. But what's wrong with that if it keeps me chugging along the road to happy destiny? I have chosen to focus on celebrating each passing year and I find that the benefits of aging far outweigh the pitfalls. It helps to have good friends and running mates who have shared our lives since grade school.

Blogger Kimberly Inskeep has a great list of "The things I love about being over fifty." I've adapted them to an additional decade, which we find is the best yet. To paraphrase her wisdom of the ages, "Regardless of our age, these things apply more broadly to the beauty of getting older in general, and when embraced can perhaps allow us to skip some stages and find joy in whatever age we happen to be."

Here are twelve advantages we've perfected after almost seven decades of experimenting:

1. Life's embarrassing moments no longer embarrass us so much, and they shift automatically to our *hilarious memories* file.

2. Our children don't expect us to be the ones who know how to work anything remotely mechanical. In fact, mine don't even expect me to operate the remote on the satellite television, which now requires two (and one is always missing).

3. Our relationships are deeper. Friends and family members who have endured our heartaches, triumphs, losses, conflicts, or just a bunch of normal Tuesdays have stuck with us for 68 years. (Bless their hearts.)

4. Glasses have become a fun fashion accessory (albeit a total necessity). They are also a handy prop for

slipping into our philosophical alter-egos, should the need arise.

5. I've learned how to make really amazing chili because I no longer feel captive to a recipe.

> • • •
>
> I have chosen to focus on celebrating each passing year and I find that the benefits of aging far outweigh the pitfalls. It helps to have good friends and running mates who have shared our lives since grade school.

6. Now that our children are all grown up, we get to spend our time in awe of the men and women they've become, instead of worrying about what they might have become.

7. I've learned the art of speaking up (or shutting up) at the appropriate times, although I need to work on the shutting up part.

8. I've found it liberating to go through drawers and closets letting go of stuff. Locks of my children's hair are not *stuff* and are more valuable than precious jewels.

9. If we overreact or get all teary-eyed during poignant moments (or coffee commercials), I can explain them away by muttering something about hormones.

10. We've let go of *balance*. It really doesn't exist. Instead, there is a willingness to let go of what doesn't matter for the sake of the things that do.

11. With time comes more great stories. We have a treasure trove of true stories, which we embellish freely.

12. Research has shown that cognitively, we are at our highest point between the ages of 40 and whatever we happen to be at the moment. I hide it well by pretending to have memory problems which I don't really have. (I've also learned to lie without guilt, especially when I'm trying to talk my way out of a speeding ticket.)

My friend Jack, who left us in December, lived by the principle that you will never see a hearse pulling a U-Haul. He was beyond generous so he could live to enjoy seeing the difference it made. I've decided to adopt his theory as my own. Anyone need a good used 15X makeup mirror? I don't have the fortitude to peer into it any longer. And those are laugh lines, not wrinkles.

Don't miss the priceless lessons of illness

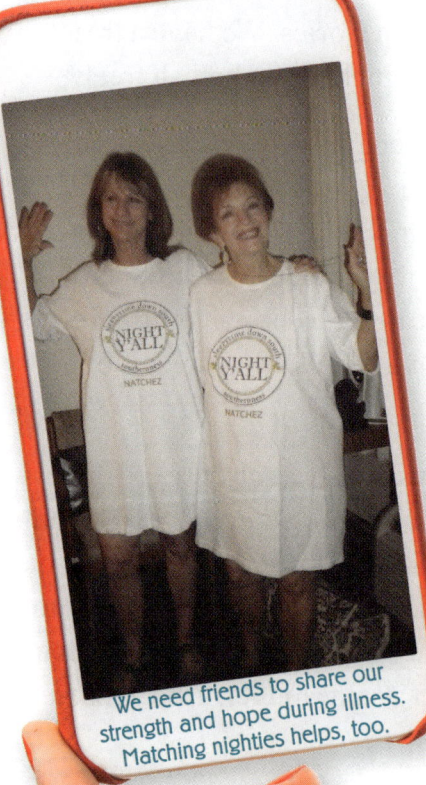

We need friends to share our strength and hope during illness. Matching nighties helps, too.

When ovarian cancer returned last October after a four month hiatus, I figured it was time to get my affairs in order. Well, not really *affairs* but you know what I mean.

I found a new doctor closer to home,

because 24 months of driving five hours for treatments had grown tiresome. I found an energetic, determined young female oncologist right here in town who promised me I would make it to my fiftieth class reunion in six months— that's all I was going for at the moment.

> • • •
>
> Cancer taught me that life isn't about playing it safe, living out our days on auto-pilot, and standing still in one spot for fear of making the wrong move. It's about experimenting, failing, succeeding, and then trying something else.

She started a revolutionary new treatment protocol which not only didn't cause many side effects but actually seemed strangely energizing. Yesterday I went for the dreaded CT scan which lit up like a Christmas tree in October with pockets of cancer lurking in lymph nodes, liver, you name it. Yesterday, the scan was as dull as a rusty nail. NO CANCER ANYWHERE!

I know I was lucky, but more than that I know I had a lot of people praying for me and I think that made all the difference. But here's the lesson in all this: I am not going to sit in my chair watching life go by while Netflix drones away on the tube. Those days are over. I'm not going to keep making excuses not to go jet skiing, zip-lining, and all the other things that make me quake in my orthopaedic shoes.

I am going to get out there and shake things up, act as weird as I please. Nobody looks stupid when they're having fun. I no longer care what anyone thinks of me, and I will be wearing my UGGS with my shorts come summer because I still won't be able to have foot surgery until the chemo drugs are gone. I am going to try new things and take risks.

Editing the local newspaper was the first big risk I took, and I fell on my face several times before figuring it out. I'm taking the train to New Orleans with my boys and we will visit our old haunts and eat the world's best cuisine and sleep on the river walk if we can find a cop to join us. Then, Marie and I are hiking the Appalachian Trail. We're taking applications for fellow hikers, but you must exhibit a degree of craziness and be at least sixty years of age.

Cancer taught me that life isn't about playing it safe, living out our days on auto-pilot, and standing still in one spot for fear of making the wrong move. It's about experimenting, failing, succeeding, and then trying something else. It's about not being at war with ourselves and wishing things were other than they are. It's about small steps toward our ever-changing dreams and getting out of our heads and into our hearts. It's about living from the soul and abandoning the façade.

We only get one shot and I'm ashamed I wasted most of mine being too timid to really live out loud. Okay, so who wants to join me in seeing how outrageously we can age and still be deliriously happy? I've always said, and believe it completely, that aging can be fabulous as long as you have someone to do it with.

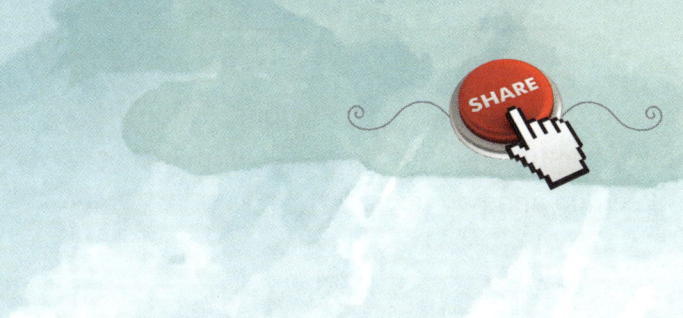

Change what I can,
but only IF I want to

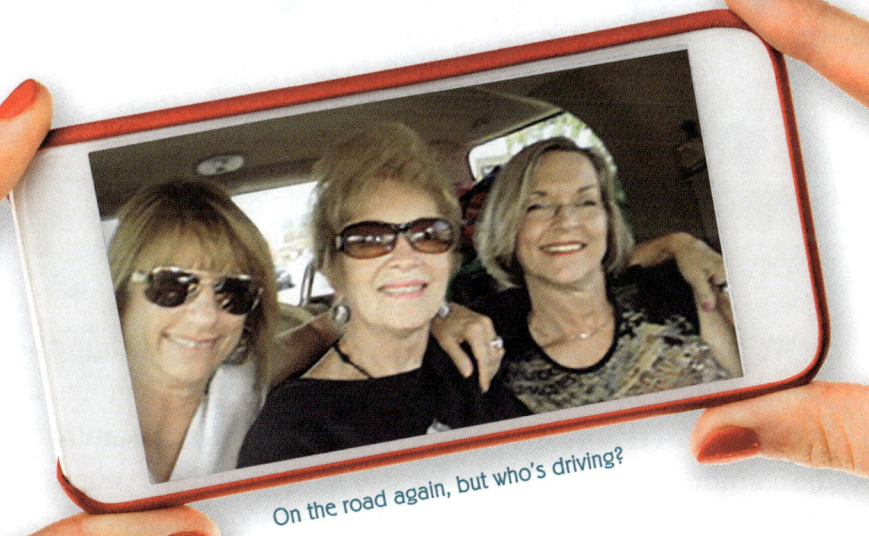

On the road again, but who's driving?

Somewhere around age 60 it became obvious to my Belligerent Boomer tribe that successful aging would require some serious recalibration of our routines and our dreams. My Numero Uno dream—other than learning a foreign language—continues to be a cabin in the woods. But I'm looking at renting one from time to time, rather than investing in another home to keep up and pay taxes on.

> • • •
>
> Someone told me once that we have to change and grow throughout life, and that we will remain stagnant if we don't get out and meet new people, read new books, and travel to new places. My gang is working on that throughout each passing year.

We also discovered that if we were still buying into the youth culture and trying to dress like twenty-somethings or people-pleasers to barter for love, friendship, and stature in the community, then we'd be wise to let it go and start our own personal revolution. My home will never be featured in *Southern Living*, and I still drive an automobile that was produced at the turn of the century (at least it was THIS century). I have a small garden in which to piddle and putter, and I never leave home without friends with whom I can laugh and kick up my heels as high as they will still go at age sixty-something.

And if I fall off the exercise/healthy living routine, I pick myself up and get back on board just as I would have done 40 years ago. As my friend Margaret Ann always says, it's no sin to fall down. It only becomes problematic when we fail to get right back up.

I, for one, am trying to break myself of that *someday* thinking—that some day when I get thin enough, rich enough, and healthy enough, I can truly begin living the life I dreamed of. Someday must become TODAY, or we're simply wasting time and taking up space and oxygen.

I've learned not to panic when working parts go on the blink without so much as a warning. That goes not only for household appliances and gadgets, but bodily parts as well. In the words of that 1950s bombshell Marilyn Monroe: "Sometimes things fall apart so other things can fall together."

Above all, I've learned to accept my current circumstances whatever they are, trusting this is where I'm meant to be for now. An old Maori proverb instructs us to "turn our face to the sun and let the shadows fall behind us." That sounds like good advice whenever things don't go according to plan. (And Mother said there would be days like this. She just didn't tell me there would be so many.)

I was attending a Sunday worship service with my dad recently when the minister concluded his thoughts with this unforgettable message: "When you come to the edge of all the light you have, and take the first step into darkness of the unknown, you must believe one of two things will happen: There will be something solid to stand upon or you will be taught to fly."

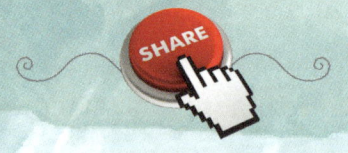

Making it up as we go along

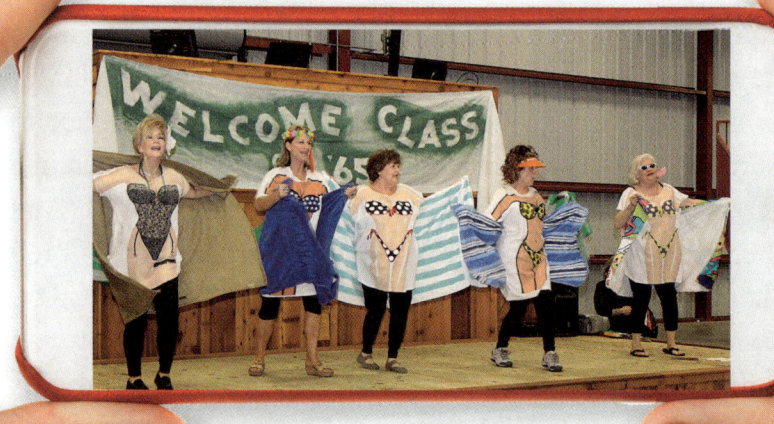

Making it up while entertaining the troops
at our 50th high school reunion

I am declaring this year officially THE YEAR OF THE BABY BOOMER in honor of those born between 1946 and 1964. Believe it or not, the babies of our generation are now in their fifties.

It's about time Boomers got some respect. We've been maligned as a selfish, greedy, statin-sucking bunch of buffoons who can't type with our thumbs (which makes texting extremely time-consuming). Hunting and pecking are our style, and as a sidebar, beware the automatic spell check. My friend Yvonne wrote her office that she was headed for a symposium and running late. Her message to her boss read, "Running late to attend to head sex." What?!?

Someone asked me just prior to New Year's if I'd made my resolutions yet. I made a sound kind of like "pufph." I've been making the same resolutions since I was old enough to write and never once kept them past January 10. What's the point?

On second thought, I think I will make some brand new resolutions befitting a good Boomer—no more droll activities like losing weight, joining a gym, giving up sugar, or getting organized. My brand new resolutions will celebrate my Baby Boomer status and target the negative changes which keep racing toward us as we dodge and duck frantically.

Here goes:

1. I will never, ever drink from a sippy cup when my boys toss me in the "home." I will slosh back martinis whenever I feel like it. (Make a note to find a trusted younger friend to sneak in the recipe and ingredients for martinis.)

2. I will never, ever wear another pair of four-inch stilettos with pointy toes, opting instead for my furry, squishy, comfy Uggs at summer, winter, and black-tie affairs.

3. I will drive by a fitness center at least once a month.

4. I will dump everything beige in my life including food and clothing, and declare orange and hot pink (preferably worn together) as the basic colors in my wardrobe.

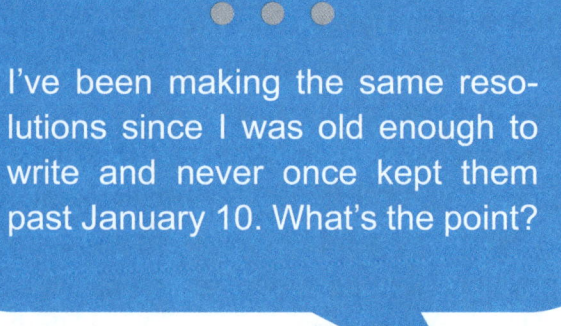

I've been making the same resolutions since I was old enough to write and never once kept them past January 10. What's the point?

5. I will stop sitting in my PJs until noon and just go back to bed.

6. I will replace the gas nozzle before driving away from the pump.

7. I'll eat more chocolate—studies show it's good for your brain and your heart.

8. I'll eat more chocolate—studies show it's good for your brain. (Uh oh, did I already list that one? I forget.)

9. I will learn how to photoshop so I can doctor the pictures I take during the many vacations my girl-friends and I enjoy at least four times a year. Turkey neck is so easily remedied.

10. I will leave my comfort zone once a month. No, scratch that. I just added it to make the list a Perfect Ten.

We are Boomers— hear us roar

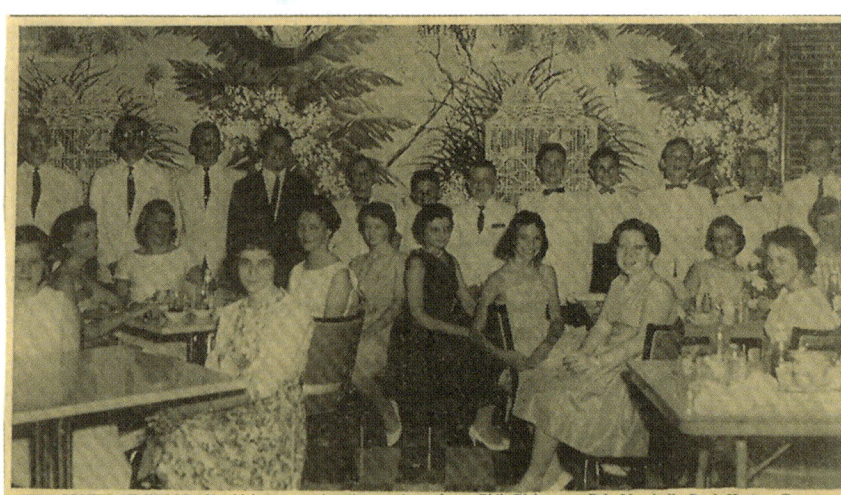

GIRL SCOUTS OF TROOP 31 which is now inactive used their remaining funds for a festive party Saturday afternoon. Shown at Mize's Restaurant where they were served a delicious luncheon are: (seated left to right) Nancy Manning, Olivia Catledge, Linda Murrah, Helen Blankenship, Ann Edwards, Emily Braddock, Carole Thompson, Linda Barton, Lucile Deas, Carole Higgins, Carolyn Blair and Julia Ann Mc-Lean. Their guests were (standing left to right): Kyle Chandler III, Alan Flowers, Doug Clark, Conley Cox, Bucky Kellogg, Phil Dickerson, Bob Marshall, Paul Hester, Tommy Robinson, Gary Florreich, Ottie Dunn and Harmon Tumlinson, Kay Cook, Norma Clark and Bobby Mac Robinson were unable to attend. The group adjourned to the John A. McLean residence for a period of games and dancing, then returned to Marshall Motel where they had a swimming party Milk shakes were served after the swim. Mrs. McLean and Mrs. Dan Thompson, former leaders, chaperoned the group. (Staff photo — Bedford)

The generation that brought us Woodstock and The Beatles isn't likely to go gently into the night. Those of us born between the years of 1946 and 1964 broke all the rules in our youth. Dare we expect this gang to go aimlessly into our Golden Years, letting them get all tarnished?

We have more senior citizens in America today than we've had at any point in history. Staying "forever young" is looking less and less likely, so we are trying to make the most of our time left on this earth.

But hey. This is what life is all about. Aging happens to every living creature and plant. It is simply a combination and culmination of many stages of development for every cell in our bodies.

Miraculously, there are days when all the pieces come together and we feel like we'll live forever—dressed to kill and feeling fabulous. On the other hand, there are days when we feel like an old shoe. I remind myself everyday of what Dr. Christiane Northrup stated in her book *Goddesses Never Age*: "The very act of thinking and behaving as if you are in your prime actually reverses the physical decline."

The prescription for being happy in both cases was offered up by Helen Keller. I try to remember it every time I feel less than satisfied with the way things are going. "When one door of happiness closes, another opens, but often we look so long at the closed door that we do not see the one that has been opened for us."

That quote has become my personal refrain as I face a changing exterior hiding the young girl who is still in here somewhere. I let her out every time two or more of us Boomers get together for an adventure. Frankly, everything has become an adventure, which often leaves us breathless. We can't wait to see what the next decade holds and how we will handle the surprises that come our way.

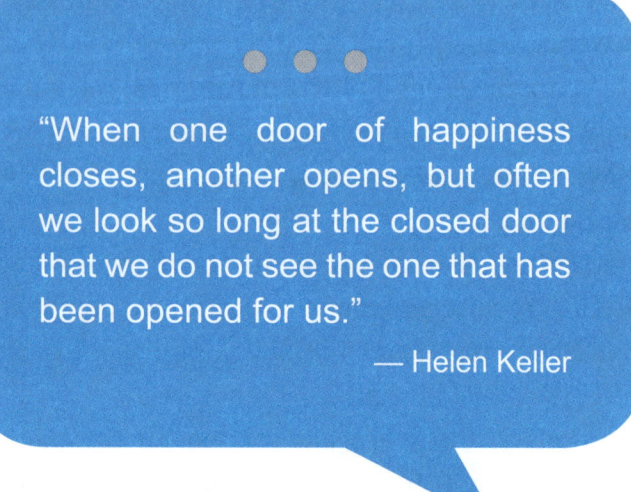

"When one door of happiness closes, another opens, but often we look so long at the closed door that we do not see the one that has been opened for us."

— Helen Keller

But I can't think about that now. I've got to map our route to Ohio to visit an old friend who has become our new friend since the class reunion. The bucket list doubled after renewing all those friendships and receiving invitations to visit faraway places. Let's get going, girls. We have a lot of ground to cover before we turn 70 and get our first tattoo.

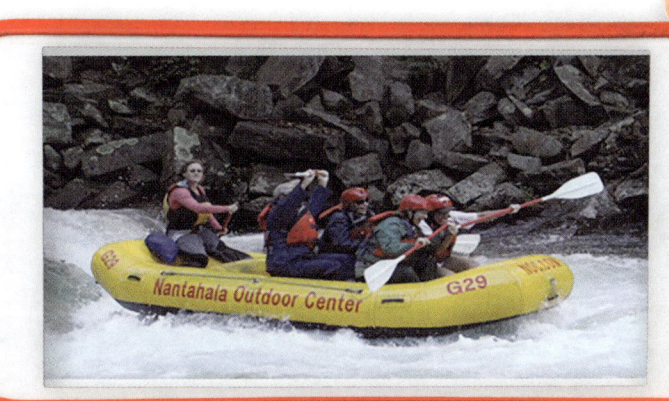

We can't wait to see what the next decade
holds and how we will handle the surprises
that come our way.